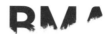

OSCEsmart

50 Medical Student OSCEs
in ENT & Opthalmology

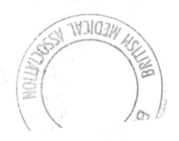

D1351187

Mr. Agbolahan Sofela

Executive Consulting Editor:
Dr. Sam Thenabadu

Ordering Information: Quantity sales. Special discounts are available on quantity purchases by corporations, associations, and others. For details, contact the publisher at the address above.

Orders by UK trade bookstores and wholesalers please visit www.scowenpublishing.com

Although every effort has been made to check this text, it is possible that errors have been made, readers are urged to check with the most up to date guidelines and safety regulations.

The authors and the publishers do not accept responsibility or legal liability for any errors in the text, or for the misuse of the material in this book.

Publisher's Cataloging-in-Publication data : OSCEsmart 50 medical student OSCEs in ENT & Opthalmology.

ISBN-10: 0-9908538-8-8
ISBN-13: 978-0-9908538-8-6

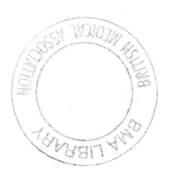

'For Verity, Pippa, Seun & Ire and of course Mum & Dad.'
Agbolahan

'For Ammi, Molly, Reuben and Rafa - I.L.Y.T.T.M.'
Sam

CONTENTS

Message from the authors

Doctors of all seniorities can remember the stress of the OSCE but even more so the stress of trying to study and practice for the OSCEs. A multitude of generic undergraduate and postgraduate resources can be found on line but quality, quantity, and completeness of content can vary. The aim of the OSCESmart editorial team is to bring together specialty focused books that have identified 50 core stations encompassing the essential categories of history taking, examinations, emergency moulages, clinical skills and data interpretation with a strong theme of communications running through all the stations.

The combined experience of consultants, registrars and junior doctors to write, edit and quality check these stations, promises to deliver content that is appropriate to reach a standard we would expect of new junior doctors entering their foundation internship years and into core training. It is important to know that these stations are all newly written and based at the level of clinical competencies we would expect from these grades of doctors. Learning objectives exist for undergraduate curricula and for the foundation years, and the scenarios are based and written around these. What they are not, are scenarios that have been 'borrowed' from any medical school.

Preparation is the key to success in most things, but never more so than for the OSCEs and a candidate that hasn't practised will soon be found out. These books will allow you to practice relevant scenarios with verified checklists to learn both content and the generic approach. The format will allow you to practice in groups with one person being the candidate, one the actor and one the examiner. Each scenario finishes with three learning points. Picture these as are three core learning tips that we would want you to take away if you had only a couple of days left to the exam. These OSCE scenarios promise to be a robust revision aide for the student looking to recap and consolidate for their exams, but equally importantly prepare them for life in clinical practice.

I am immensely proud of this OSCESmart series. I have had the pleasure of working with some of the brightest and most dynamic young clinicians and educators I know, and I am sure you will find this series covering the essential clinical specialties a truly robust and invaluable companion in those stressful times of revision. I must take this opportunity to thank my colleagues for all their hard work but most of all to thank my wonderful wife Molly for her unerring love and support and my sons Reuben and Rafael for all the joy they bring me.

Despite the challenging times the health service finds itself in, being a doctor remains a huge privilege. We hope that this OSCESmart series goes some way to help you achieve the excellence you and your patients deserve.

Best of luck, Dr Sam Thenabadu

Introduction to OSCESmart 50 OSCEs OSCES in ENT:

Medical students and doctors generally find OSCEs terrifying, fact! This could be because ENT and ophthalmology are often not covered in as much detail as other specialties in medical school, with most students' only experience being a day spent in an outpatient clinic or in theatres watching an interesting case. This often causes a situation where students study only with an aim to get through the ENT and ophthalmology sections of their exams, and not necessarily to master clinical skills within these specialties that they can apply to their day to day clinical practice. This book aims to address that.

The initial challenge in writing this book was getting the balance right; between having cases with concise messages relevant for studying for the OSCEs, and more detailed information that can be applied in real clinical situations. The finished product gets this balance just right.

Most of the cases require three students to the; patient/actor (occasionally, an additional actor will be necessary), examiner and the candidate. I cannot emphasize enough the importance of being involved in each of these roles as the book gives insight into what the examiner expects of you, the key symptoms (from the Actors point of view) you'll expect to see with certain diseases and presentations, and of course the candidate's point of view.

This book covers a great deal of ENT & Ophthalmology presentations and also covers in detail, advanced communication skills in a dedicated section, all in just 50 cases. Most of the cases here detail clinical scenarios I and the co-authors have all come across at some point, and you are more than likely to come across too, not only in your OSCEs, but also in real clinical practice.

Working through all the cases in this book will not only make you prepared for OSCE stations in ENT or Ophthalmology, but will also make you more confident handling the common clinical scenarios encountered whilst working in these specialties.

Good luck with your studies, exams and future medical careers.

I would like to take this opportunity to say a big thank you each and everyone of my co-authors (Chris, Neil, Kush, Pedro, Gareth and Mihiar) for the hard graft put into delivering what is a very high standard & quality OSCE book. I know I harassed you every single step of the way, chasing our weekly deadlines; your effort is genuinely appreciated.

Finally, I want to acknowledge some of the truly amazing and inspiring teachers I've had over the years (Richard Gullan, Daniel Walsh, Ranj Bhangoo, Mo Faruque, Nick Thomas, Richard Selway, Iannois Panagopoulos, Jacek Adamek, Sanj Bassi, Nilesh, Jose, Meriem, Ahilan, Jig, Kostas, Haru, and many more whose names I've to omit to avoid filling up the first 200 pages of this book), Alysha (the best clinical partner anyone can wish for), and one of the best consultants I've ever had the pleasure of working with; Sam Thenabadu.

Mr Agbohalan Sofela,
November 2016

About the Authors

Mr Agboholan Sofela

BSc(Hons) MBBS MRCS (Eng)
Specialty Trainee in Neurosurgery, UK

Agbolahan Sofela completed his undergraduate medical training in King's College Medical School in 2013. During his period studying at King's, he completed an intercalated anatomy BSc degree, which further fanned his interest in pursuing a career in surgery, in particular neurosurgery, thanks to dissection projects involving the CNS and PNS.

He completed his Foundation training in the South Thames Foundation school in London. He spent a year as a Core surgical trainee in the London deanery, during which time he completed his Royal College of Surgeons membership exams. After this he applied for, and was appointed the South West Deanery's Neurosurgical trainee.

Academically, he has won several awards for research, teaching, professionalism and contributions towards medical societies; both at undergraduate and postgraduate levels. He has published several papers in Peer reviewed journals, and given numerous oral and poster presentations at regional, national and international conferences.

He is a champion of medical education, and has been involved with teaching at all levels of his medical training, culminating in an award of recognition of his 'Outstanding achievement in teaching', bestowed on him by the Kent & Canterbury Hospital, UK.

He has had the luxury of being taught and influenced by truly inspiring teachers and it is easy to see why he has such a great passion for teaching; a cycle he hopes to continue.

Dr Sam Thenabadu

MBBS MRCP DRCOG DCH MA Clin Ed FRCEM MSc (Paed) FHEA

Consultant Adult & Paediatric Emergency Medicine
Honorary Senior Lecturer & Associate Director of Medical Education

Sam Thenabadu graduated from King's College Medical School in 2001 and dual trained in Adult and Paediatric Emergency Medicine in London before being appointed a consultant in 2011 at the Princess Royal University Hospital. He has Masters degrees in Clinical Medical Education and Advanced Paediatrics.

He is undergraduate director of medical education at the King's College NHS Trust and the academic block lead for Emergency Medicine and Critical Care at King's College School of Medicine. At postgraduate level he has been the Pan London Health Education England lead for CT3 paediatric emergency medicine trainees since 2011. Academically he has previously written two textbooks and has published in peer review journals and given numerous oral and poster presentations at national conferences in emergency medicine, paediatrics, medical education and patient quality and safety.

He has an unashamed passion for medical education and strives to achieve excellence for himself, his colleagues and his patients, hoping to always deliver this through an enjoyable learning environment. Service delivery and educational need not be two separate entities, and he hopes that those who have had great teachers will take it upon themselves to do the same for others in the future.

Co- Authors

Dr Christopher Ashton MBBS MSc.
Ophthalmology ST1 KSS

Mr Mihiar Sami Atfeh - MRCSed, DOHNS, MD.
Specialty Doctor & Honorary University Fellow – Plymouth Hospitals NHS Trust & Plymouth University.

Mr Kush Bhatt MBBS Bsc MRCS.
ST3 Neurosurgery South West Peninsula Deanery

Dr. Neil Bowley MChem (hons), BMBS, PhD.
ST3 Ophthalmology South West Peninsula Deanery

Mr Gareth Lloyd BMBS BMedSci (Hons) MRCS DOHNS.
Specialty Registrar (StR) Otorhinolaryngology, London

Dr Pedro Santos Jorge MBBS LMD MMedEd.
Foundation trainee 2, London

Section 1

Ear Cases

Case 1

Candidates instruction:

You are the ENT Foundation doctor and have been asked to take the initial history from a 15 year old boy presenting with right sided ear pain. Take a concise history and summarise your findings back to the team.

After 6 minutes the examiner will stop you and ask you to summarise back your findings, suggest your management plan and answer some direct questions.

Examiner's instruction:

This is a scenario of a teenager complaining of otalgia. It is a relatively short history in an otherwise fit and well patient.

The main focus of this station is for the candidate to realise that there is an acute on chronic component of ENT presentations, especially at the patient's age and in ear presentations. The candidate should also demonstrate an understanding of the relationship between pharyngitis and otalgia and vice versa.

After 6 minutes, please stop the candidate and ask:

"Please summarise your findings and discuss how you would like to investigate and manage this patient."

Actors instruction:

You are a 15 year old boy with a 3 day history of right ear pain following a particularly long swimming session. The pain is worse on touching or pulling on the ear, you tend to suffer from recurrent ear infections for which you currently have a grommet in situ. There is an offensive thin green discharge from the ear with intermittent bleeding but no redness, or any other obvious skin changes.

You've had a sore throat with large 'glands' inside your mouth (tonsils) for 2 weeks but are not quite sure of the relevance; at this point, ask the candidate if they feel there is a connection. If they say no, challenge them on this

Mention that you are currently having try-outs for the British junior swimming Olympic team, and cannot afford to stop swimming. Expect empathy when a link is made between swimming and your ear pathology, and relent at this point.

Case 1 Task:	Achieved	Not Achieved
Introduces themselves & clarifies who they are speaking to and relationship to child		
Elicits history from parent/child in a concise manner		
Takes a structured pain history using e.g. SOCRATES		
Specifically asks about:		
Redness		
Swelling		
Temperature/other skin changes		
Pruritis		
Discharge - Color, smell, consistency		
Associated pharyngitis		
Associated headaches		
Previous infections		
Deafness		
Dizziness/balance problems		
Asks about CN V, VII, IX symptoms		
Mastoid tenderness		
Asks about birth & past medical/surgical/drug history		
Checks allergy status		
Explores Ideas, concerns, and expectations		
Demonstrates good rapport and empathy with the patient throughout		
Relays a concise summary to the examiner		
Examiner's Global Mark	/5	
Actor / Helper's Global Mark	/5	
Total Station Mark	/30	

Learning points:

- Main differentials here include: **infection, cellulitis, tonsillitis. Being able to take a good structured pain history is important for most surgical history taking stations; practice this. SOCRATES is one of many ways of systematically taking a pain history

  Site
  Onset
  Character
  Radiation
  Associated symptoms
  Timing (course of pain)
  Exacerbating/alleviating factors
  Severity

- In this station, it is important to realize that pain can be referred along the CN V tracts (dental), or the oropharynx (CN IX), so ask specifically for symptoms pertinent to these cranial nerves.

- It is also important to note the important points that can be gained for communication skills (listening, rapport, empathy and question asking – always start histories with open questions)

Case 2

Candidates instruction:

You are the Emergency Department Foundation doctor and have been asked to take the initial history from a 6 year old boy presenting with 'muffled' hearing. Take a history and summarize your findings as you would when referring to the ENT registrar on-call.

After 6 minutes the examiner will stop you and ask you to summarise back your findings, suggest your management plan and answer some direct questions.

Examiner's instruction:

This is a scenario of a child complaining of left sided hearing impairment. He is otherwise well, up to date with his vaccinations, and cooperative throughout the entire history, though the candidate should demonstrate an ability to ask specific questions in order to get the full history from the child.

The main focus of this station is for the candidate to focus his history taking around the 2 most common causes of paediatric ear presentations; foreign body and infection

After 6 minutes, please stop the candidate and ask:

"Please summarise your findings and discuss how you would like to investigate and manage this patient."

Actors instruction:

You are a 6 year old boy with a 2 day history of left sided muffled hearing. Onset of symptoms was right after playing in the playground with other kids. The child is normally very inquisitive and tends to put things either into his various orifices (this particular info should only be provided if asked directly).

The child can still hear sounds and whispers, but very distorted in the left ear. Also complains of associated intermittent left otalgia, minimal discharge from the ear (slightly blood stained and non-offensive), and a 'weird' fullness in the ear.

If asked directly, the child can reveal that whilst playing with his friend, they wondered if a piece of plasticine will fit in their respective ears

Case 2 Task:	Achieved	Not Achieved
Introduces self & clarifies who they are speaking to and relationship to child		
Elicits history from parent/child in a concise manner		
Ascertains extent of hearing loss (whisper, soft words etc)		
Specifically asks about: Onset of symptoms Rate of onset (Insidious/rapid) Unilateral or bilateral symptoms Temperature/other skin changes Discharge (Color, smell, consistency) Associated pharyngitis Associated headaches Previous infections Deafness Dizziness/balance problems History of foreign bodies in bodily orifices Mastoid tenderness		
Asks about birth & past medical/surgical/drug history		
Checks allergy status		
Explores Ideas, concerns, and expectations		
Demonstrates good rapport and empathy with the patient throughout		
Relays a concise summary to the examiner		
Examiner's Global Mark	/5	
Actor / Helper's Global Mark	/5	
Total Station Mark	/30	

Learning points:

- The main differentials here include foreign body and an infection. These are the most common causes of ear presentations considering the age of the boy in this scenario.

- It can be difficult getting a detailed history from children, so It is important to take time to elicit what information the child may be able to provide, to get a strong collateral history and then to ask direct questions.

- It is also important to note the soft communication points (listening, rapport, empathy and question asking) are especially important in this statio.

Case 3

Candidates instruction:

You are a Foundation doctor doing a rotation at a GP practice. The next patient is complaining of a left sided otorrhoea. Please take a concise history and summarise your findings.

After 6 minutes the examiner will stop you and ask you to summarise back your findings, suggest your management plan and answer some direct questions.

Examiner's instruction:

This is a scenario of a 35 year old man presenting with a 5 day history of discharge from the left ear. Please assess the candidate specifically on how concise the history is. The candidate should appreciate that unilateral otorrhoea in an adult should be taken seriously as it can indicate an infection, or more rarely, head and neck malignancies.

The candidate should very clearly ascertain if the symptoms are acute, chronic, or associated with signs/symptoms of malignancy.

After 6 minutes, please stop the candidate and ask:

"Please summarise your findings and discuss how you would like to investigate and manage this patient."

Actors instruction:

You are a 35 year old man with a 5 day history of discharge from the left ear with associated tenderness when the pinna is pulled, tenderness over the bony prominence below/behind the ear, and muffled hearing on the left side
You have never had this problem before, and besides having your adenoids and tonsils removed as a child, are otherwise fit and well.

If asked directly, volunteer that; the discharge is offensive, yellow, sometimes blood stained, is persistent, often leaves yellow crusts on your pillow and associated with headaches.

You smoke 40 cigarettes a day and have done so for 20 years. If the candidate asks you if there is a family history of ear problems or family history of medical problems in general, ask them if they want to know about any specific conditions. Essentially, unless asked directly, do not volunteer the information that your dad and his dad died of a large cancer inside the nose
If the candidate does not mention cancer, you should act very worried about the possibility of this being cancer. Ask the candidate of it is possible for cancers in the nose to cause ear problems

Case 3 Task:	Achieved	Not Achieved
Introduces self & clarifies who they are speaking to		
Specifically asks the following about the discharge: Color & Smell Consistency (thick, thin, serous, etc) Is it exacerbated by positioning? Timing (intermittent/constant) Unilateral or bilateral Does the discharge alleviate any headaches		
Screens for infective process: Pain/otalgia (ear, mastoid, peri-auricular area) Erythema (location and extent)/other skin changes Temperatures/rigors etc Previous infections		
Screens for symptoms associated with malignancy: Unintentional weight loss/loss of appetite Night sweats Lethargy/general malaise Associated nasal congestion Rhinorrhea, post nasal drip		
Asks about past medical/surgical/drug history & allergies		
Explores Ideas, concerns, and expectations		
Demonstrates good rapport and empathy with the patient throughout		
Relays a concise summary to the examiner		
Examiner's Global Mark	/5	
Actor / Helper's Global Mark	/5	
Total Station Mark	/30	

Learning points:

- Possible differentials for this station are acute otitis media, chronic suppurative otitis media, chronic otitis media, or in the context of trauma, CSF otorrhoea

- Recognizing the relationship between nasopharyngeal malignancies and ear presentations is important re compression of the Eustachian tubes

- Patients with significant family histories of malignancy can be very anxious about the possibility of them having the same. You will gain points in an OSCE and credibility in clinical life for being reassuring, confident and give an aura of a doctor that can be trusted by your patients

Case 4

Candidates instruction:

You are the Emergency Department Foundation doctor and have been asked to take the initial history from a 66 year-old woman presenting with 'muffled' hearing. Take a history and summarize your findings as you would when referring to the ENT registrar on-call.

After 6 minutes the examiner will stop you and ask you to summarise back your findings, suggest your management plan and answer some direct questions.

Examiner's instruction:

This is a scenario of a woman complaining of left sided hearing impairment. As a child, she was treated for ADHD, had several multiple skin lesions excised by a dermatologist (neurofibromas), is currently being worked up for a possible optic sheath glioma, but is otherwise fit and well. She is grossly deaf on the left side and requires the candidate to direct conversations to the contralateral side, whilst talking loudly and clearly.

The candidate should be able to realise earlier on in the consultation that this is a possible Neurofibromatosis 1 (NF1) diagnosis, and should tailor the questions in such a way

The station is directed towards history taking only and therefore the candidate should be reminded of that should he/she try to carry out a clinical examination.

After 6 minutes, please stop the candidate and ask:

"Please summarise your findings and discuss how you would like to investigate and manage this patient."

Actor instructions:

You are a 66 year old woman who has been troubled for the past three months with progressive left sided hearing difficulties. You went in to see the GP this morning because you had a severe headache this morning, and since then, the left side of your face is now numb with some sagginess of the muscles – you are worried about a stroke.

The deafness came on gradually over the past year, and has gotten worse over the past 3 months to the extent that you make people speak to you on your right side, and now find yourself getting told off by your husband for talking too loudly because you cannot hear how loudly you're speaking

You have a past history of ADHD (as a child), you have had several skin 'bumps' removed by a dermatologist, and have an appointment to see an ophthalmologist in a week's time because of an abnormal growth seen at the back of your right eye last time you went for a repeat prescription for your glasses.

You have no drug allergies, and besides your prescription skin cover makeup (for 'weird skin marks') you take no regular medications

You do not smoke, and only drink socially.

There is a family history of strokes, hypertension and breast cancer

You are a retired lawyer, enjoy your classical music and generally live a life of leisure

You are particularly worried about having a stroke, and you express this concern on several occasions during the consultation. You only relent when the candidate reassures you that whilst a stroke is a possibility, it is highly unlikely to explain your symptoms

18

Case 4 Task:	Achieved	Not Achieved
Introduces self & clarifies who they are speaking to		
Specifically asks the following about the hearing loss Side Onset (sudden/insidious) & time frame of symptom progression Recent trauma to the head/skull base? Recent viral/bacterial infections (URTI)? Associated otorrhoea, skin changes, otalgia Associated dizziness, vertigo, tinnitus, headaches Associated CN V (hemi-facial sensory changes) and CN VII (hyperacusis and facial muscle paresis) symptoms		
Recognizes the possibility of NF1 as a diagnosis and screens specifically for them by checking for: MSK abnormalities such as bony dysplasias, bowing of long bones Cutaneous abnormalities (café au lait patches, neurofibromas) Neurological development disorders (ADHD, learning difficulties) Family history of NF1 Mental disorders (depression, anxiety etc) Other neurological diseases (seizures, other CNS/PNS tumours)		
Asks about past medical/surgical/drug history & allergies		
Family and social history		
Clearly demonstrates a knowledge of how NF1 present from the type of questions asked		
Explores Ideas, concerns, and expectations and demonstrates good rapport and empathy with the patient throughout		
Relays a concise summary to the examiner		
Suggests other reasonable differentials		
Examiner's Global Mark	/5	
Actor / Helper's Global Mark	/5	
Total Station Mark	/30	

Learning points:

- The main differential to exclude here is a vestibular schwannoma/acoustic neuroma. Others include presbyacusis, tympanic membrane perforations, obstruction of the ear canal, dislocation of the ossicular chain, otosclerosis, tympanosclerosis, Meniere's disease, etc

- In this station, it is important to realize that the constellation of symptoms such as unilateral deafness, mental disorders (ADHD), optic nerve tumours, and café au lait patches are highly indicative of an acoustic neuroma so the questions you ask the patient must reflect this realization. If a tumour is large enough, it can also compress the 7th and 5th cranial nerves, and can cause facial hemi-sensory changes with associated paresis, and in some cases, headaches.

- Know about the diagnostic criteria for Neurofibromatosis 1 and 2, the genetic aetiology, genetic inheritance patterns, and the management options. Note that any possible new tumour/cancer diagnosis has to be discussed sensitively with patients, especially in this case where there is a significant implication on the patient's offspring.

Case 5

Candidates instruction:

You are a Foundation doctor doing a rotation in the emergency department. The next patient is a 6 year old boy who has been sent to hospital by the school nurse with a bleeding left ear. Please take a concise history and summarise your findings as you would when referring to the ENT registrar on-call.

After 6 minutes the examiner will stop you and ask you to summarise back your findings, suggest your management plan and answer some direct questions.

Examiner's instruction:

This is a scenario of a 6 year old boy presenting acutely with blood from the left ear.

Asses the candidate specifically on how concise the history is. The candidate should appreciate that unilateral bloody-otorrhoea in a child is most likely to be trauma or foreign body related, and as such, the questions asked whilst the candidate takes the history should be along these lines.

Ensure the candidate understands the range of differentials with this particular presentation in a paediatric setting, in order of how common they are, i.e. trauma and foreign body being most common in a child at school, followed by infection (acute or chronic) and less commonly, malignancies. If the candidate describes malignancy as a top differential, challenge them on this and emphasize the importance of mentioning the commoner differentials first.

The candidate should suggest an ear (with a comprehensive ENT) examination + +/- toileting as the first line management in an emergency department setting.

After 6 minutes, please stop the candidate and ask:

"Please summarise your findings and discuss how you would like to investigate and manage this patient.

Actors instruction:

Two actors may be required for this station; one is the patient, the other is the mother

You are a 6 year old boy with bleeding from the left ear. You were playing in the playground when your best friend inserted a pencil into your left ear. The bleeding started as soon as you removed the pencil.

The ear was incredibly painful initially, but since the school nurse gave you some Calpol, you feel much better. The blood was bright red, there was a lot of it, bled for about 15 minutes, but thankfully, the bleeding has stopped.

Since the bleeding stopped, you have noticed that your hearing from the left side is muffled, and you have a funny sensation in your left ear, best described as 'something poking your ear hole'.

You have no temperatures, no pus from the ear, no neck swelling, no redness of the external ear or canal, etc, no signs of an infection

Your mum can confirm that you are have suffered in the past with multiple ear infections on the right side, have had a grommet inserted into the right side, and are now partially deaf on the right side. The fact that you may potentially lose hearing on the left side is extremely distressing for your mum, and when your mum asks if there is a chance your left ear/sided hearing may be permanently impaired, you also get very distressed.

Mum can also confirm that you are otherwise fit and well, up to date with vaccinations, and besides the steroid ear drops you take for the right ear, you do not take any other regular medications, and have no allergies
**Mother:

Ask specifically for the possibility of your child being permanently deaf on the left side. If the candidate attempts to deflect the question, you can get increasingly aggressive with the questioning until you get a clear answer. If the candidate claims that there is no chance of this, you can get very distressed and request to speak to a more senior doctor than a FY2. If the candidate suggests that permanent impairment is a possibility, then point out that this may mean that your child is permanently deaf (bilaterally); expect a clear demonstration of empathy at this point.

Case 5 Task:	Achieved	Not Achieved
Introduces self & clarifies who they are speaking to		
Specifically asks the following about the discharge: Color Consistency (thick, thin, serous, etc) Events around onset of bleeding - trauma, foreign body (in a playground, swimming, fighting, etc) Timing (intermittent/constant)		
Screens for infective process: Pain/otalgia (ear, mastoid, peri-auricular area) Erythema (location and extent)/other skin changes Temperatures/rigors etc Previous infections		
Screens for other symptoms associated with bloody otorrhoea: Check for any palpable masses/lesions in the ear canal Hearing loss Tinnitus Dizziness and vertigo Facial palsy		
Checks for previous episodes of similar presentations		
Asks about past medical/surgical/drug history and allergies		
Checks the child's social circumstances, i.e. lives with siblings, no supervision at home, and generally checks that the child's home environment is safe		
Explores Ideas, concerns, and expectations		
Demonstrates good rapport and empathy with the patient throughout		
Relays a concise summary to the examiner		
Examiner's Global Mark	/5	
Actor / Helper's Global Mark	/5	
Total Station Mark	/30	

Learning points:

- Possible differentials for this station are foreign body, trauma, acute otitis media, chronic suppurative otitis media, chronic otitis media, Eustachian tube dysfunctions, or more rarely, the first presentation of a malignancy (ear canal squamous cell carcinomas, polyps, etc)

- Most paediatric ear presentations that involve blood are either due to trauma or an infection. In the context of a young child in a playground, trauma (including foreign bodies) should be the top of the differential list. It is rare for patients in this age group to present with ear bleeding as a first sign of a pertinent malignancy.

- In this particular scenario, there is a history of pre-existing contralateral hearing impairment. Dealing with the patient/parents has to be done in an exceptionally sensitive manner. When discussing the possibility of permanent damage to the left ear in this case, this should be done sympathetically and sensitively but ensuring there is no ambiguity in the message you convey.

Case 6

You are the ENT Foundation doctor and have been asked to see a patient presenting with right sided ear pain. Take a **brief history, examine** the patient and **present** your findings whilst suggesting potential differentials and the immediate management plan (for your top differential) to your consultant.

After 6 minutes the examiner will stop you and ask you to summarise back your findings, suggest your management plan and answer some direct questions.

Examiner's instruction:

This is a scenario of a woman who presents with otalgia. It is a 1 week history of pain, with associated mastoid swelling and tenderness. The patient is a poorly controlled Non-Insulin dependent diabetic.

The main focus of this station is for the candidate to realise that when examining the ear, inspection of the external ear and surrounding areas is key. This scenario describes a patient with mastoiditis, who has presented with a soft tender red lump over the mastoid process, but with the severe otalgia being the main distracting symptom.

It is expected that the candidate is able to identify the mastoid abnormality and direct the questions in this manner, i.e an infective process stemming for the mastoid.

The candidate should also be able to carry out be a concise ear exam, and should suggest at the end that they will like to carry out a full ENT exam (including the oropharynx), a full examination of the face to include the skin overlying the facial sinuses and other bony prominences. The candidate should also mention that they will like to check the bedside clinical observations, routine bloods (including inflammatory markers), and to suggest either an ultrasound of the lump or more preferable a CT scan of the head to include a bony window and the sinus. It is also appropriate for the candidate to suggest formal audiometric testing in light of the 'muffled' hearing on the symptomatic side.

After 6 minutes, please stop the candidate and ask:

"Please summarise your findings and discuss how you would like to investigate and manage this patient."

Examination findings:

Pt appears well, nil distress
HR 65
BP 125/88mmHg
Temp 37.8°C
RR 15
Blood sugar (capillary) 26mmmol

Ear appears mildly red, with a moderately large red swelling noted over the mastoid process. Nil skin breakdown and no obvious discharge
The pinna and the mastoid swelling are both mildly warm to touch, tender on palpation, with the pain worse when the pinna is pulled inferiorly and in an anterior/posterior direction

There is a minimal yellow-green offensive smelly serous discharge within the ear canal. There is also a soft 'buggy' brown debris. This is not adherent to the skin lining the ear canal. The tympanic membrane is intact, and appears grossly normal

Hearing is reported as 'slightly muffled' on the right side. No indication for a formal Weber's Rinne's test in the context of this station, but this should be suggested as appropriate further tests when summarizing to the examiner.

The oropharynx is normal on gross examination

Actors instruction:

You are an 86 year old woman with a 6-day history of right ear pain. The pain is worse on touching or pulling on the ear, and you have tried simple analgesia to no effect.

You report no problems with your hearing, but on examination, you find that sounds (especially whispers) sound more muffled on the right side. You have not noticed any discharge from the ear, have no previous ear infections, no dizziness or balance problems, no recent trauma to the ear, and the pain does not radiate anywhere else besides the ear itself and the mastoid process.

You do have a moderately sized lump over the bone behind your ear which has increased in size over the past 2 weeks. This lump is soft, red, warm to touch and tender to touch (though not as bad as the ear). You saw your GP about this lump a week ago and he started you on a broad spectrum antibiotic, but you don't quite know why.

Pulling on your 'ear lobe' downwards makes the pain worse. You jump in pain when anything (including the otoscope) is inserted into the ear canal, but you will tolerate the exam only once the candidate offers you analgesia.

No abnormalities inside the mouth/oropharynx on examination

You are a heavy smoker, obese, a poorly controlled 2 diabetic, take no other medications regularly besides the antibiotic prescribed by your GP and Insulin, have no allergies, and are a social drinker.

Case 6 Task:	Achieved	Not Achieved
Introduces self & clarifies who they are speaking to		
History:		
Takes a structured pain history using e.g. SOCRATES (checks for radiation down to the neck, up towards the temple, mastoid process, jaw, etc)		
Specifically asks for other symptoms: Redness, skin changes (around the ear) Temperature spikes Headaches Discharge (color, smell, consistency) Previous infections/recent trauma Deafness, dizziness or balance (gait) problems		
Asks about past medical/surgical/drug history & allergy status (specifically checks for a history of diabetes mellitus)		
Examination:		
Inspects the external ear, and surrounding areas Palpates the external ear and surroundings, feeling for temperature changes or any palpable lumps Makes a point of pulling on the pinna in several directions to replicate the otalgia Palpates for mastoid tenderness Performs an otoscopy and comments on the ear canal, and tympanic membrane as appropriate Grossly assesses hearing (whisper test) Inspects the oropharynx looking for obvious signs of pathology in the posterior oropharynx Palpates for any cervical lymphadenopathy		
Demonstrates good rapport and empathy with the patient throughout, and explores their ideas, concerns, and expectations		
Elicits history from patient in a concise manner		
Relays a concise summary to the examiner		
Examiner's Global Mark	/5	
Actor / Helper's Global Mark	/5	
Total Station Mark	/30	

Learning points:

- The main differentials here include: infection (malignant otitis externa, acute otitis externa, acute otitis media, mastoiditis, cellulitis), malignancies of the ear canal or skull base, etc.

- Note that there is a well-documented strong correlation between T2DM (diabetes) and mastoiditis, and as such, your history and examination should reflect that you are aware of this fact, especially in this patient's age group.

- Being able to take a good structured pain history is important for most surgical history taking stations; practice this. SOCRATES is one of many ways of systematically taking a pain history.

Case 7

Candidates' instruction:

You are a Foundation doctor doing a rotation at a GP practice. The next patient is complaining of a rash around his right ear. Please take a concise history and summarise your findings

After 6 minutes the examiner will stop you and ask you to summarise back your findings, suggest your management plan and answer some direct questions.

Examiner's instruction:

This is a scenario of a 24 year old man presenting with a 3 day history of redness around his right ear. Please assess the candidate specifically on how concise the history is. The candidate should appreciate that erythema in an adult can indicate an infection, bacterial or viral.

The candidate should very clearly ascertain if the symptoms are acute, chronic, or associated with dysfunction of ear/pain.

After 6 minutes, please stop the candidate and ask:

"Please summarise your findings and discuss how you would like to investigate and manage this patient."

Actors instruction:

You are a 24 year old man with a 3 day history of erythema with associated tenderness when the pinna is pulled, tenderness over the tragus, and muffled hearing on the left side. You have never had this problem before and are otherwise fit and well. If asked directly, volunteer that; hearing is normal, no discharge from the ear itself and you have had an intermittent fever.

If the candidate asks you if there is no family history of ear problems or family history of medical problems in general, ask them if they want to know about any specific conditions.

If the candidate does not ask you about your hearing, you should enquire if this is going to make you deaf as you are worried because you are a musician.

Case 7 Task:	Achieved	Not Achieved
Introduces self & clarifies who they are speaking to		
Specifically asks the following about the rash: Site Spreading Itchiness Skin broken Precipitating event (bite/scratch) Is it raised (can you feel it under your fingers)		
Screens for infective process: Pain/otalgia (ear, mastoid, peri-auricular area) Area feel warm Fevers Previous infections		
Screens for symptoms associated with infection: Recent URTI Night sweats Lethargy/general malaise Associated nasal congestion Rhinorrhea, post nasal drip		
Asks about past medical/surgical/drug history & allergies		
Explores Ideas, concerns, and expectations		
Demonstrates good rapport and empathy with the patient throughout		
Relays a concise summary to the examiner		
Examiner's Global Mark	/5	
Actor / Helper's Global Mark	/5	
Total Station Mark	/30	

Learning points:

- Possible differentials for this station are cellulitis, herpes zoster, varicella zoster, perichondritis, other causes of rash; urticarial, atopic

- Recognizing that a rash in a dermatomal distribution may represent varicella zoster and needs to be treated with aggressive steroid therapy

- It is good to ascertain what is concerning the patient regarding his hearing and the possible implications to his future career.

Case 8

Candidates' instruction:

You are a Foundation doctor doing a rotation in the Emergency Department. The next patient is complaining of dizziness. Please take a concise history and summarise your findings

After 6 minutes the examiner will stop you and ask you to summarise back your findings, suggest your management plan and answer some direct questions.

Examiner's instruction:

This is a scenario of a 30 year old woman presenting with a 1 week history of dizziness. Please assess the candidate specifically on how concise the history is. The candidate should appreciate that dizziness in an adult can be peripheral (related to ear) to central (CNS).

The candidate should very clearly ascertain if the symptoms are acute, chronic, or associated with dysfunction of ear.

After 6 minutes, please stop the candidate and ask:

"Please summarise your findings and discuss how you would like to investigate and manage this patient."

Actors instruction:

You are a 30 year old woman with a 1 week history of dizziness, particularly when getting up from bed. This is associated with nausea and you have vomited twice.

You have never had this problem before and only have a past medical history of IBS. If asked directly, volunteer that; hearing is normal, no discharge from the ear itself and you have had some ringing in your ears.

If the candidate asks you if there is no family history of ear problems or family history of medical problems in general, ask them if they want to know about any specific conditions.

If the candidate does not ask you about your concerns, you should enquire if this is going to stop you driving as you don't think you can drive safely but are worried about picking your children from school.

Case 8 Task:	Achieved	Not Achieved
Introduces self & clarifies who they are speaking to		
Specifically asks the following about the dizziness: When it occurs and previous episodes? What makes it worse / better Does the room spin? Associated Visual disturbance? Any blackouts? Any nausea?		
Screens for causes: Recent URTI Headaches Any neurological symptoms (facial weakness / numbness) Previous dizziness		
Screens for associated symptoms: tinnitus hearing loss unilateral or bilateral symptoms Any medications which may precipitate dizziness URTI symptoms		
Asks about past medical/surgical/drug history & allergies		
Explores Ideas, concerns, and expectations		
Demonstrates good rapport and empathy with the patient throughout		
Relays a concise summary to the examiner		
Examiner's Global Mark	/5	
Actor / Helper's Global Mark	/5	
Total Station Mark	/30	

Learning points:

- Possible differentials for this station are BPPV, labrynthitis, Meniere's Disease, Vestibular Schwannoma, vestibular migraines

- Recognising that unilateral signs (tinnitus / hearing loss) associated with dizziness may indicate pathology affecting the vestibular cochlear nerve (vestibular schwannoma)

- It is good to ascertain what is concerning the patient regarding driving and the possible implications to her life. Allowing time for this exploration of her ideas, concerns and expectations is well worth while as much of the pertinent history may also be concurrently elicited.

Case 9

Candidates' instruction:

You are a Foundation doctor doing a rotation in GP. The next patient is complaining of ringing in his ears. Please take a concise history and summarise your findings.

After 6 minutes the examiner will stop you and ask you to summarise back your findings, suggest your management plan and answer some direct questions.

Examiner's instruction:

This is a scenario of a 54 year old man presenting with a 1 month history of tinnitus. Please assess the candidate specifically on how concise the history is. The candidate should appreciate that tinnitus in an adult can be bilateral or unilateral.

The candidate should very clearly ascertain if the symptoms are acute, chronic, or associated with dysfunction of ear.

After 6 minutes, please stop the candidate and ask:

"Please summarise your findings and discuss how you would like to investigate and manage this patient."

Actors instruction:

You are a 54 year old man with a 1 month history of intermittent tinnitus. This is associated with dizziness, nausea and reduced hearing.

You have never had this problem before and have a past medical history of ischaemic heart disease. If asked directly, volunteer that; hearing is reduced, no discharge from the ear itself and you have had some dizziness.

If the candidate asks you there is family history of ear problems and heart disease, but you are unsure of what the disease is.

If the candidate does not ask you about your concerns, you should enquire if this is going to get worse.

Case 9 Task:	Achieved	Not Achieved
Introduces self & clarifies who they are speaking to		
Specifically asks the following about the ringing: When it occurs? What makes it worse / better Intermittent / persistent? Hearing disturbance Does it keep the patient awake? Any nausea?		
Screens for causes: Recent URTI Headaches Any neurological symptoms (facial weakness / numbness) Previous ringing		
Screens for associated symptoms: dizziness hearing loss unilateral or bilateral symptoms Any medications which may precipitate dizziness URTI symptoms		
Asks about past medical/surgical/drug history & allergies		
Explores Ideas, concerns, and expectations		
Demonstrates good rapport and empathy with the patient throughout		
Relays a concise summary to the examiner		
Examiner's Global Mark	/5	
Actor / Helper's Global Mark	/5	
Total Station Mark	/30	

Learning points:

- Possible differentials for this station are labrynthitis, Meniere's Disease, Vestibular Schwannoma.

- Recognising that unilateral signs (tinnitus / hearing loss) associated with dizziness may indicate a sinister pathology affecting the vestibular cochlear nerve (vestibular schwannoma)

- It is important in this station to ascertain which of the symptoms is most concerning for the patient; deafness tends to be the most debilitating symptoms as it has a huge impact on normal day to day life. Most patients merely find tinnitus an annoyance.

Case 10

Candidates instruction:

You are the Foundation doctor working at a GP practice. Your next patient complaints of a lump by his left ear. Please examine this lump and present your findings and differentials to the examiner.

After 6 minutes the examiner will stop you and ask you to summarise back your findings, suggest your management plan and answer some direct questions.

Examiner's instruction:

This is a scenario of a 30 year old man presenting with a 1 year history of a lump behind the left ear.

Please assess the candidate specifically on how fluent the lump examination is. The candidate should very clearly assess for tenderness prior to touching the lump

After 6 minutes, please stop the candidate and ask:

"Please summarise your findings and discuss how you would like to investigate and manage this patient."

Examination findings:

The lump is behind the left ear, it is fixed to the skin but not to any underlying structures

There is no pain

There is no mastoid tenderness

There is no erythema

Examination of the canal is NORMAL

Actors instruction:

You are a 30 year old male attending a GP practice. For the past year you have noticed a lump behind your left ear, it's normally not painful but occasionally can be and sometimes it leaks fluid which is yellow and occasionally blood stained. As it has persisted you have come to the GP to find out what it is.

You are otherwise well and have never had any hearing problems before.

Examination findings:

The lump is behind the left ear, it is fixed to the skin but not to any underlying structures

There is no pain

There is no mastoid tenderness

There is no erythema

Examination of the canal is NORMAL

Case 10 Task:	Achieved	Not Achieved
Introduces self & clarifies who they are speaking to		
Briefly explains examination and obtains consent		
Asks about any hearing problems		
Asks about pain		
Assessment of lump Assessment of erythema and warmth		
Places lump between 2 fingers and attempts to mobilise it		
Assesses if fixed skin		
Assess if fixed to underlying structures		
Assess if compressible		
Checks if pulsatile		
Looks for punctum		
Tests for mastoid tenderness		
Repeats procedure on other ear		
Identifies abnormality		
Elects to use otoscope to check canal		
Checks contralateral ear first		
Ensures that lump does not extend into canal		
Asks to check for regional lymphadenopathy		
Demonstrates good rapport with the patient throughout		
Demonstrates empathy appropriately		
Relays a concise summary to the examiner		
Interpreters findings adequately		
Examiner's Global Mark	/5	
Actor / Helper's Global Mark	/5	
Total Station Mark	/30	

Learning points:

- All lumps should be assessed for adherence to underlying structures, a punctum, overlying skin changes, shape, consistency and colour.

- All head and neck regional lymph nodes should be assessed, and the patient should be asked about any other swellings found in the axilla, groin or a sense of abdominal swelling that could indicate organomegaly

- Must ask about pain BEFORE examining. Both in the OSCE and clinical practice, patients will cooperate and assist examinations far better if their pain is enquired about, acknowledged and dealt with as early as possible.

Case 11

Candidates instruction:

You are the Foundation doctor working at a GP practice. Your next patient complaints of reduced hearing in the **right ear**.

Examine this patient's hearing.

After 6 minutes the examiner will stop you and ask you to summarise back your findings, suggest your management plan and answer some direct questions.

Examiner's instruction:

This is a scenario of a 30 year old man presenting with a 1 year history of a lump behind the left ear.

Please assess the candidate specifically on how fluent the lump examination is. The candidate should very clearly assess for tenderness prior to touching the lump

After 6 minutes, please stop the candidate and ask:

"Please summarise your findings and discuss how you would like to investigate and manage this patient."

Examination findings:

With the tuning fork on the forehead (Weber's test) you will hear **LOUDEST** on the **RIGHT** ear – lateralising to the *RIGHT*

When examining the **LEFT** ear (Rinne's test) the tuning fork sounds **LOUDEST** in **FRONT** of the ear (AC) than **BEHIND** the ear (BC).

When examining the **RIGHT** ear (Rinne's test) the tuning fork sounds **WORSE** in **FRONT** (AC) of the ear then **BEHIND** the ear (BC).

Patient has a **Right sided conductive hearing loss

Actors instruction:

You are a 56-year-old female attending a GP practice. For the past 40 years, you have cleaned your ears regularly with cotton buds after showering in spite of being advised against it. This morning you have cleaned your ears as usual but your hearing from the **RIGHT** ear became worse afterwards. You are otherwise well and have never had any hearing problems before. There is no blood or discharge.

Examination findings:

With the tuning fork on the forehead (Weber's test) you will hear **LOUDEST** on the **RIGHT** ear – lateralising to the *RIGHT*

When examining the **LEFT** ear (Rinne's test) the tuning fork sounds **LOUDEST** in **FRONT** of the ear (AC) than **BEHIND** the ear (BC).

When examining the **RIGHT** ear (Rinne's test) the tuning fork sounds **WORSE** in **FRONT** (AC) of the ear then **BEHIND** the ear (BC).

Patient has a **Right sided conductive hearing loss

Case 11 Task:	Achieved	Not Achieved
Introduces self & clarifies who they are speaking to		
Briefly explains examination and obtains consent		
Asks about any hearing problems		
Chooses appropriate tuning fork		
Rinne's test		
Handles tuning fork appropriately and makes it vibrate		
Positions vibrating tuning fork over the mastoid bone		
Asks if patient can hear any sound		
Positions vibrating tuning fork in front of the ear		
Asks if patient can hear any sound		
Asks where tuning fork sounded the loudest		
Repeats procedure on other ear and is able to Identify the abnormality		
Weber's test		
Handles tuning fork appropriately and makes it vibrate		
Positions vibrating tuning fork over the forehead		
Asks if can hear sound on both ears and if so if it's the same		
Identifies that there is abnormality		
Identifies a Right sided conductive hearing loss		
Demonstrates good rapport with the patient throughout		
Demonstrates empathy appropriately		
Relays a concise summary to the examiner		
Interpreters findings adequately		
Examiner's Global Mark	/5	
Actor / Helper's Global Mark	/5	
Total Station Mark	/30	

Learning points:

- Weber's and Rinne's should be interpreted together

- Weber's symmetrical in normal hearing
    - In conductive hearing loss, *lateralises* towards affected side
        - i.e: loudest in the affected side
    - In sensorineural hearing loss, *lateralises* away from affected side
        - i.e: loudest in the contralateral side

- Rinne's tests air conduction (AC) *versus* bone conduction (BC)
    - AC•BC in both sides in normal hearing
    - AC•BC in sensorineural hearing loss on affected side
    - BC•AC in conductive hearing loss on affected side

Case 12

Candidates instruction:

You are the surgical foundation year doctor attached to the emergency department and have been asked to assess a patient presenting with discharge from the **right** ear.

Examine the patient's hearing whist he is waiting for a CT head.

After 6 minutes the examiner will stop you and ask you to summarise back your findings, suggest your management plan and answer some direct questions.

Examiner's instruction:

This is a scenario of a 27 year old man presenting acutely with right sided otorrhoea following trauma.

Please assess the candidate specifically on how fluent the examination is. The candidate should very clearly assess for tenderness prior to touching the patient

The station should take 8 minutes in total, with a warning bell 2 minutes prior to the end, and the last 1 minute for a clear summary and presentation of the examination findings and differentials

Examination findings:

You feel there is water in the ear, especially if you lean forwards, and you have also noticed a small bruise behind the right ear.

With the tuning fork in on the forehead (Weber's test) you will hear **LOUDEST** on the **LEFT** ear – lateralizing to the *LEFT*

When examining the each ear separately (Rinne's test) the tuning fork sounds **LOUDEST** in **FRONT** of the ear (AC) than **BEHIND** the ear (BC) on both ears.

Actors instruction:

You are a 27-year-old male attending the emergency department after being involved in a fight outside a pub the night before. You can't remember what happened exactly because you were drunk. Today you noticed that you're not hearing very well from your *right* ear, and you also had to wipe a small amount of pink liquid from the *right ear-lobe*. There is some pain if you press around it.

You are otherwise well and have never had any hearing problems before.

Examination findings:

You feel there is water in the ear, especially if you lean forwards, and you have also noticed a small bruise behind the right ear.

With the tuning fork in on the forehead (Weber's test) you will hear **LOUDEST** on the **LEFT** ear – lateralizing to the *LEFT*

When examining the each ear separately (Rinne's test) the tuning fork sounds **LOUDEST** in **FRONT** of the ear (AC) than **BEHIND** the ear (BC) on both ears.

Case 12 Task:	Achieved	Not Achieved
Introduces self & clarifies who they are speaking to		
Briefly explains examination and obtains consent		
Makes a point of inspecting the ear and around it (Battle's sign)		
Chooses appropriate tuning fork		
Rinne's test		
Handles tuning fork appropriately and makes it vibrate		
Positions vibrating tuning fork over the mastoid bone		
Asks if patient can hear any sound		
Positions vibrating tuning fork in front of the ear		
Asks if patient can hear any sound		
Asks where tuning fork sounded the loudest		
Repeats procedure on other ear		
Identifies abnormality		
Weber's test		
Handles tuning fork appropriately and makes it vibrate		
Positions vibrating tuning fork over the forehead		
Asks if can hear sound on both ears and if so if it's the same		
Identifies abnormality		
Identifies possible traumatic skull base injury		
Demonstrates good rapport with the patient throughout		
Relays a concise summary to the examiner		
Interpreters finding adequately		
Examiner's Global Mark	/5	
Actor / Helper's Global Mark	/5	
Total Station Mark	/30	

Learning points:

- When considering hearing loss in the context of trauma, consider both conductive and sensorineural hearing loss patterns.

- A skull base fracture along the path of CNVII can cause an injury to the nerve.

- Accumulation of blood/CSF in the auditory system (internal/external auditory meatus) can also simulate a conductive hearing loss

Case 13 - Data interpretation

You are a foundation doctor attending your first ENT clinic. The consultant running the clinic is very keen on teaching, and he has arranged a data interpretation teaching session for you. This is your chance to impress the consultant with your knowledge.

You have 8 minutes for this session, but will get a warning bell 2 minutes prior to the end. Please use this remaining time to collect your thoughts and discuss any other important points you will like to cover.

Part 1 – Audiograms

Audiogram 1:
i.   Interpret the following audiogram and suggest one possible diagnosis.
ii.   Explain to the examiner how to perform Rinne's test.
iii.   Explain to the examiner what the expected result of performing Rinne's test on this ear would be, presuming the other ear has normal hearing thresholds.?

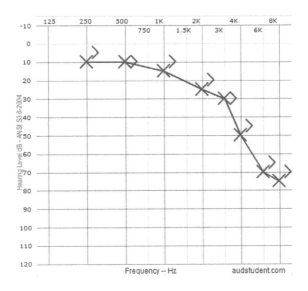

Audiogram 2:

i. Interpret the following audiogram and suggest one possible diagnosis.
ii. Explain to the examiner how to perform Weber's test.
iii. Explain to the examiner what the expected result of performing Weber's test on this patient would be, presuming the other ear has normal hearing thresholds.

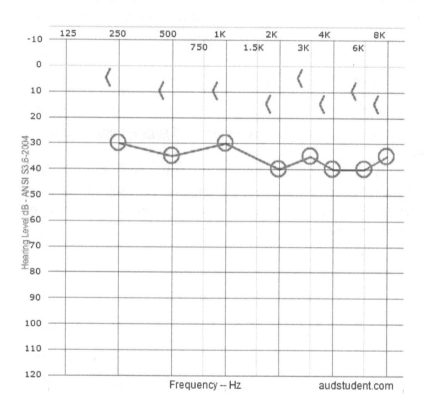

Audiogram 3:

i.　Interpret the following audiogram and suggest a possible diagnosis.

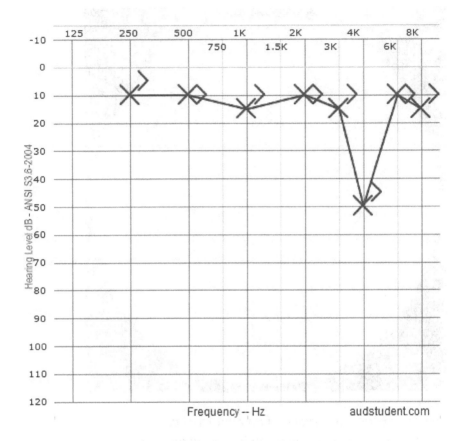

Part 2 - Otoscopy.

Otoscopy 1:

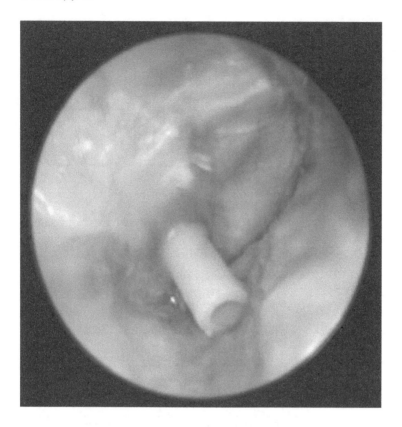

This is an otoscopic image of an abnormal tympanic membrane
i.   What surgical intervention has occurred here?

Otoscopy 2:

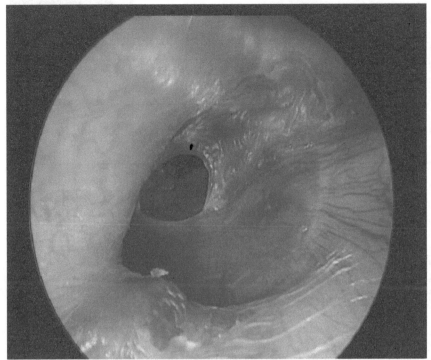

This is an otoscopic image of an abnormal tympanic membrane

i.   What pathology is shown here?

Case 13 Task:	Achieved	Not Achieved
Audiogram 1:		
Interpretes the audiogram as showing a sensorineural hearing loss in the left ear		
Identifies that the higher frequencies are affected		
Identifies presbycusis as a likely underlying diagnosis, but allow any condition that may cause a sensorineural hearing loss such as a vetibular schwannoma		
Rinne's Test: Hold a vibrating 512Hz tuning fork on the mastoid until the subject can no longer hear it and move to with 1-2cm of the auditory canal and ask the patient if they can still hear the ringing		
Rinnes will be positive (AC>BC)		
Audiogram 2:		
Interpretes the audiogram as showing a conductive hearing loss (CHL) in the right ear		
Identifies any reasonable cause of a CHL including: canal atresia, wax/FB impaction, perforated tympaninic membrane, middle ear effusion, otosclerosis as a likely underlying diagnosis		
Weber's Test: Hold a vibrating 512Hz tuning fork on the centre of the forehead (or central incisors) and check for lateralization.		
Webers will lateralize to the affected (right) side		
Audiogram 3:		
Identifies audiogram shows hearing thresholds for the left ear		
Identifies a sensorineral hearing loss at 4000Hz		
Identifies the likely cause is noise induced hearing loss.		
Rinnes will be negative (AC<BC)		
Webers will lateralize to the affected (right) side		
Otoscopy 1:		
Identifies a ventilation tube (allow T-tube or grommet)		
Otoscopy 2:		
Identifies a tympanic membrane perforation		
Assesses and interprets the audiograms/otoscopy images systematically		
Examiner's Global Mark	/10	
Total Station Mark	/30	

Learning points:

- Pure Tone Audiograms (PTA) display the hearing thresholds at a range of frequencies. It relies on the subject pressing a button when they hear the noise presented either via a headphone down the ear canal (air conduction, AC) or via a vibrating source against the skull (bone conduction, BC).
It is essential to learn the symbols:
X = AC left ear
] or **>** = BC left ear
O = AC right ear
[or **<** = BC right ear ear
Any symbol accompanied by a downwards arrow denotes that the threshold is unrecordable

- Weber's and Rinne's tuning fork tests are easy to perform and it helps to use both tests to interpret your findings accurately. In a normal hearing patient Weber's test will be heard equally or centrally. Weber's will lateralize towards a unilateral CHL and away from a unilateral SNHL. Rinne's test is considered positive (normal) if AC is perceived louder than BC.

- Orientate yourself to otoscopy photographs by identifying the lateral process of the malleus. It always points anteriorly and therefore you can tell that photograph 1 is of a right ear. The tympanic membrane (TM) is often translucent or may have a perforation which reveals the middle ear structures. Be aware of which structures lie behind each quadrant of the TM.

Section 2

Nose & Sinus Cases

Case 14

Candidate instructions:

A 58 year old female patient presents to the emergency department with a three-day history of epistaxis. As the Foundation doctor who is covering ENT overnight, you were asked by the ED consultant to take a full history from the patient. The patient had nasal packing carried out by the paramedics who transported her to the hospital. On arrival you are informed that the patient has no active further bleeding, and has a normal cardiovascular assessment.

After 6 minutes the examiner will stop you and ask you to summarise back your findings, suggest your management plan and answer some direct questions.

Examiner's instructions:

This is a scenario of a recurrent epistaxis in a female patient who is being treated with oral antibiotics by her GP for a UTI (urinary tract infection). The patient has a medical history of hypertension and a metallic AVR (aortic valve replacement) but is otherwise fit and healthy. The patient takes anti-hypertensives and warfarin regularly and has no allergies.

The station is directed towards history taking only and therefore the candidate should be reminded of that should he/she try to carry out a clinical examination. The candidate should be assured that the patient is cardiovascularly stable, is packed with no active bleeding, and has an IV access secured.

After 6 minutes, please stop the candidate and ask:

"Please summarise your findings and discuss how you would like to investigate and manage this patient."

Actor instructions:

You are a 58 year old woman who has been troubled for three days with recurrent nose bleeds. You were diagnosed a week ago by your GP with a urinary tract infection and were given antibiotics (Co-Amoxiclav) to treat that. The infection was diagnosed as you were experiencing burning and frequency in your water works, and was confirmed with a dip-stick test by your GP. There is no recent history of trauma, nose surgery, nose picking. You bruise easily but otherwise have no personal or familial bleeding history.

You have 20 years history of high blood pressure. You were diagnosed many years ago with aortic valve stenosis (narrowing) and for that you had 3 years ago a metallic valve replacement. You regularly take Ramipril and Atenolol (for your blood pressure) and Warfarin (a blood thinner to stop blood clots formation on your metallic). You otherwise are fit and healthy, take no other medications, and have no allergies. You have never smoked, rarely drink alcohol, and work at the post office.

The nosebleeds have been recurring for three days but never occurred before. They come from the right nostril, but sometimes they happen from both nostrils and drip at the back of your throat. The bleeding episodes usually last for less than 20 minutes, but tonight your nose bleed failed to stop. Therefore you called 999 and the ambulance crew packed your nose to stop the bleeding. You currently have pressure pain in your nose and face (the nurse had just given you oral morphine for this), but otherwise have no other symptoms and no active bleeding.

Case 14 Task:	Achieved	Not Achieved
Introduces self & clarifies who they are speaking to		
Asks if the patient prefers the presence of relatives / nurses and if they are happy for the encounter to take place in the current environment		
Clarifies if the patient has (and expresses willingness to address) any pain / discomfort / needs methodically (e.g. "SOCRATES")		
Asks about the development of bleeding (onset / frequency / duration)		
Asks about the location(s) of bleeding (right / left / anterior / posterior)		
Asks about nasal symptoms (obstruction, rhinorrhea, anosmia, post nasal drip, facial headaches)		
Asks about any history of trauma / surgery to area / nose picking		
Asks about history of recent upper respiratory tract infections		
Asks about any history of using anticoagulants		
Ask about history of hypertension		
Ask about history of bleeding disorders		
Explores the presence of general symptoms (night sweats / fever / weight loss / recurrent infection)		
Ask about past and recent medical / surgical history		
Checks drug history		
Checks allergy status		
Checks social and family history		
Elicits history in a concise and clear manner		
Explores the patient's and relative's ideas, concerns, and expectations		
Demonstrates good rapport and empathy with the patient and relatives throughout the encounter		
Relays a concise summary to the examiner		
Examiner's Global Mark	/5	
Actor / Helper's Global Mark	/5	
Total Station Mark	/30	

Learning points

- Epistaxis is commonly caused by trauma (including nose picking), iatrogenic (anticoagulants, surgery, cocaine), and bleeding disorders. The severity and onset of the haemorrhage define the most effective management (conservative, medical, or surgical). Therefore, thorough history taking is crucial in order to define the likely cause(s) and best management plan.

- Epistaxis patients are commonly under significant stress due to pain and anxiety. This usually causes tachycardia, a rise in blood pressure and subsequently a higher risk of bleeding. Therefore the patient's anxiety and pain must be promptly assessed and addressed, preferably through a methodical manner (e.g. SOCRATES).

- A calm, confident, and reassuring approach by the doctor can play a key role in addressing the patient's anxiety. Good rapport with the patient and relatives also assists the doctor in establishing a clear coherent history and gaining the patient's trust. OSCEs that have global marks reflect this and can swing a station one way or the other.

Case 15

Candidates instruction:

You are the Foundation doctor working in a GP practice. Your next patient complaints of a poor sense of smell. Take a full **history** from this patient.

After 6 minutes the examiner will stop you and ask you to summarise back your findings, suggest your management plan and answer some direct questions.

Examiner's instructions:

The station is directed towards history taking only and therefore the candidate should be reminded of that should he/she try to carry out a clinical examination.

After 6 minutes, please stop the candidate and ask:

"Please summarise your findings and discuss how you would like to investigate and manage this patient."

Actors instruction:

You are a 56 year-year-old male builder and the reason why you came to see the doctor is because your wife has been nagging you for ages that you can't smell properly! You've never had a good sense of smell and always put it down to smoking so you don't really see the point of coming in at all.

You concede that it's probably getting worse but you're not bothered about it too much. The only thing that concerns you is that you're finding it increasingly hard to take part in the local pub's annual cider tasting competition because your sense of taste has deteriorated as well. You frequently have colds and a blocked nose even in summer but always put is down to the fact that you work outdoors.

You suffer from asthma and take the blue inhalers on occasions. You have high blood pressure for which you take amlodipine and diabetes for which you take metformin. Your mates complain that you snore very loudly when you travel with them to the construction sites!

Case 15 Task:	Achieved	Not Achieved
Introduces self & clarifies who they are speaking to		
Elicits history from patient in a structured and concise manner		
Asks about onset of symptoms		
Asks about associated signs or symptoms such as pain, nasal discharge, blocked nose, difficulty breathing, snoring		
Asks about specific conditions such as sinusitis, rhinitis		
Asks about neurological signs/symptoms: Seizures Headaches Visual problems		
Asks about changes in mood, or personality		
Asks about changes on sense of taste		
Asks about facial trauma		
Asks about drug history/allergy status		
Asks about recreational drugs, namely snorting		
Family history		
Asks about smoking/alcohol history		
Asks about occupation		
Asks about past medical/surgical		
Explores Ideas, concerns, and expectations		
Demonstrates good rapport with the patient throughout		
Demonstrates empathy appropriately		
Relays a concise summary to the examiner		
Examiner's Global Mark	/5	
Actor / Helper's Global Mark	/5	
Total Station Mark	/30	

Learning points:

- Anosmia can be a subtle symptom and difficult to assess so often patients don't value it too much. However, its causes can be significant, and includes frequently missed pathologies such as head and neck/intracranial malignancies.

- Note that head and neck malignancies have a high prevalence in patients of oriental origin

- Following a thorough ENT examination, Investigations for anosmia include (and are not limited to) CT heads +/- contrast, CT sinuses, MRI head (including sinuses), Naso-endoscopy, etc.

Case 16

Candidates instruction:

You are the Foundation doctor working in GP practice. Your next patient complaints of nasal discharge. Take a full **history** from this patient

After 6 minutes the examiner will stop you and ask you to summarise back your findings, suggest your management plan and answer some direct questions.

Examiner's instructions:

The station is directed towards history taking only and therefore the candidate should be reminded of that should he/she try to carry out a clinical examination.

After 6 minutes, please stop the candidate and ask:

"Please summarise your findings and discuss how you would like to investigate and manage this patient."

Actors instruction:

You are a retired 72-year-old joiner who presents with nasal discharge. This has been going on for many months and you initially thought it was just a cold but you never seem to get rid of it completely. The discharge is usually clear but you're concerned that lately is often yellowish and bloody. The nose is occasionally blocked, curiously always on the left side. Your left eye is often watery. There is no pain but you feel there is some fullness around the eyes. You noticed that clothes seem to be a bit looser than they used to be but you're happy about it as you needed to lose some weight anyway. Your sense of smell is terrible but it has always been like that. There is no history of trauma.

You had asthma and hay fever as a child but that is long gone now. You used to smoke 20-a-day but stopped five years ago when you had a heart attack. You consider yourself in relatively good health and apart from the heart attack and a bit of arthritis of the left knee you are OK. You're happy that clothes seem to be a bit looser as of late because you needed to lose some weight. You take aspirin, Ramipril, Bisoprolol and Simvastatin. On Friday nights you usually go to the pub and have a couple of pints of lager.

Case 16 Task:	Achieved	Not Achieved
Introduces self & clarifies who they are speaking to		
Elicits history from patient in a structured and concise manner		
Asks about onset of symptoms		
Asks about the discharge (color, thickness, smell, bloody)		
Asks about associated signs or symptoms such as pain, blocked nose, difficulty breathing, snoring		
Asks about other local signs/symptoms (headaches, vision/eye problems, swallowing)		
Asks about systemic symptoms (loss of appetite, weight loss, night sweats, malaise)		
Asks about changes on sense of smell		
Asks about facial trauma		
Asks about drug history and allergies		
Family history		
Asks about social history - smoking/alcohol history and occupation		
Asks about past medical/surgical, specifically conditions: Sinusitis (Allergic) rhinitis Nasal polyps		
Explores Ideas, concerns, and expectations		
Demonstrates good rapport with the patient throughout		
Demonstrates empathy appropriately		
Relays a concise summary to the examiner		
Identifies the need to refer to secondary care via the 2 week wait suspected cancer pathway.		
Examiner's Global Mark	/5	
Actor / Helper's Global Mark	/5	
Total Station Mark	/30	

Learning points:

- Polyps are the most common (benign) neoplastic cause of nasal discharge so it is important to always specifically check for a history of polyps as patients can disregard this as a relevant past medical history

- Malignancies of the facial complex/skull base are rare and often present late as their signs/symptoms can be subtle or absent until advanced stages of disease. It's important to be screen for red flags and not dismiss nasal discharge as a common cold or rhinitis/sinusitis. Note that there is a high incidence of head and neck (especially nasopharyngeal) malignancy in patients of 'oriental' origin. This includes Japan, China, etc

- Don't forget that common things are common and patients will commonly present with chronic sinusitis. Please rule this out before pursuing the malignancy route as a diagnosis.

Case 17

Candidates instruction:

You are the Foundation doctor working at a GP practice. Your next patient complaints of headaches. Take a full **history** from this patient

After 6 minutes the examiner will stop you and ask you to summarise back your findings, suggest your management plan and answer some direct questions.

Examiner's instructions:

The station is directed towards history taking only and therefore the candidate should be reminded of that should he/she try to carry out a clinical examination.

After 6 minutes, please stop the candidate and ask:

"Please summarise your findings and discuss how you would like to investigate and manage this patient."

Actors instruction:

You are a 43-year-old male. For the last couple of weeks you've been having headaches and facial pain. It's mostly on the left side of the head, extending to the forehead, between the eyes and down to the left cheek. Your upper teeth are now aching and you find this odd because you recently had a dental checkup. It all started about three weeks ago when you had a bit of a runny nose and a sore throat and never really got better. Pain is dull and you feel your face to be "full".

It's worse in the morning and when you lean forwards. You feel awful and your nose is blocked. When you blow it there is yellowish thick discharge. You've tried paracetamol over-the-counter but don't seem to do much good. You don't have any visual disturbances, painful or a red eye, nausea & vomiting.

Similar events happened in the past but not this bad nor this long. There is no history of trauma. The whole thing is affecting your job (you work in a pet shop) because you can't concentrate and deal with clients. On top of everything, your partner has been complaining of you having bad breath!

You used to smoke about 10 cigarettes/day but stopped years ago and had hay fever as a child. You don't have any allergies.

Case 17 Task:	Achieved	Not Achieved
Introduces self & clarifies who they are speaking to		
Elicits history from patient in a structured and concise manner		
Takes a structured pain history using e.g. SOCRATES		
Asks about precipitating/aggravating factors/duration		
Asks about associated symptoms such as: Visual disturbances Photophobia Painful/red eye		
Asks about fever/neck stiffness		
Asks about nasal blockage/laterality		
Asks about discharge		
Asks about previous occurrences		
Asks about facial trauma		
Asks about drug history including nasal decongestants and drug allergies		
Family history		
Asks about social history - smoking/alcohol history and occupation		
Asks about past medical/surgical history focusing on head & neck procedures		
Explores Ideas, concerns, and expectations		
Demonstrates good rapport with the patient throughout		
Demonstrates empathy appropriately		
Relays a concise summary to the examiner		
Examiner's Global Mark	/5	
Actor / Helper's Global Mark	/5	
Total Station Mark	/30	

Learning points:

- Main differentials here include: **trauma, sinusitis (mastoid, ethmoid, etc). Being able to take a good structured pain history is important for most surgical history taking stations; practice this. SOCRATES is one of many ways of systematically taking a pain history

- Headaches can have a wide ranging etiology, it's important to ask broad-based questions and elicit appropriate red flags.

- Remember that the sinuses are also likely culprits for headaches, especially when associated with flu like symptoms, are generalized, and include the face

Case 18

Candidates instruction:

You are the Foundation doctor on a GP placement. Your next patient is Herman, a 60 year old man who according to your records was seen last week with mild sinusitis, but before this hadn't been seen for 15 years:

'Patient phoned 0800, given same day appointment – c/o right eye swelling'

Take a **short history and examine** this patient presenting with unilateral facial swelling.

After 6 minutes the examiner will stop you and ask you to summarise back your findings, suggest your management plan and answer some direct questions.

Examiner's instructions

When the patient is being examined give the appropriate clinical findings if the candidate performs the correct examination technique or describes what they would like to do to elicit a clinical sign.

Ask the candidate to summarize their findings and offer a differential diagnosis with a management plan.

After 6 minutes, please stop the candidate and ask:
"Please summarise your findings and discuss how you would like to investigate and manage this patient."

Examination findings:

Observations
Comfortable at rest on room air
Resp. rate 20, SpO2 98% on room air
Pulse 90, BP 128/79 Capillary refill time 3 seconds, Warm peripheries
38.5°C

Inspection
Both upper and lower eyelids of the right eye are swollen and erythematous but not swollen shut.
Chemosis
Proptosis
Looking up patient's nose – mucoid discharge from right nostril

Palpation
Both lids tender to palpation

Examination of external eye
Ocular motility – restricted and painful on the right eye
Visual acuity 6/12 right 6/6 left
Pupillary testing: equal and reactive

Actors instruction:

You are Herman a 60 year old man with a 12 hour history of swelling around the right eye.

You noticed a small area of redness and swelling in the upper eyelid last night. This has progressed to involve both upper and lower lids this morning and has seemed to get worse between making the appointment and seeing his GP.

Patient's eye has become very bloodshot and the white part has become swollen. 'it looks like a jelly like substance is around the eye'.

Patient has been suffering double vision this morning. It is relieved by closing either eye.The vision isn't as good as it usually is in the right eye.Patient has developed pain around the eye and forehead, and this is made worse by reading or by looking around and moving the eye.

Patient has been suffering with a stuffy, blocked nose for the past week or so, and has been feeling under the weather. Today though patient feels much worse, and is feeling uncharacteristically poorly.

Herman has no past medical history and is incredibly fit for his age, running the London marathon in under 4 hours two months ago. Wears glasses for reading and is colour blind. No regular medications. No known allergies. You take a multivitamin.

You live with your wife. A lifelong non-smoker, you work as an accountant, patient drives.No relevant family history, children and grandchildren are fit and well.

Your primary concern is that you will have to be admitted to hospital. You had your tonsils out as a child and it was a horrific experience, making you phobic of doctors and hospitals. You only came today to the GP because your wife forced you.

Case 18 Task:	Achieved	Not Achieved
Introduces self & clarifies who they are speaking to		
Washes / Gels hands		
History of presenting complaint. Specifically: Onset & elicits rapid progression of symptoms		
Associated ocular symptoms. Specifically: Change in vision & diplopia		
Headache history: SOCRATES		
Past medical and ophthalmic history		
Checks for any current medications and checks allergy status		
Examination – Basic observations		
Examination – Inspect Notes swelling of both lids of the right eye, Notes chemosis, Notes proptosis, Looks in up nose		
Examination - Palpation		
Examination – Ocular motility Restricted and painful		
Examination – Visual Acuity – states that intends to measure visual acuity. Prompt candidate to move on, informing the candidate that if they performed VA testing it would be found to be decreased in the right eye to 6/12		
Examination – assessment of pupils Direct / consensual / RAPD		
Explores Ideas, concerns, and expectations		
Demonstrates good rapport and empathy with the patient		
Relays a concise summary to the examiner		
Offers differential diagnosis Orbital cellulitis		
Management plan (3 marks) Admit to hospital Intravenous antibiotics Scan required		
Examiner's Global Mark	/5	
Actor / Helper's Global Mark	/5	
Total Station Mark	/30	

Learning points:

- The patient has signs and symptoms suggestive of orbital cellulitis. Recognition that the patient has a potentially life threatening illness, and that prompt action is required is the key knowledge requirement for this station.

- Orbital cellulitis is occasionally preceded by a coryzal illness and can be rapidly progressive. Complications include: Sepsis, extra-orbital spread of infection, abscess formation, cavernous sinus thrombosis, and loss of vision due to central retinal artery occlusion / compressive optic neuropathy.

- Treatment of orbital cellulitis is with high dose intravenous antibiotics. Imaging of the head is mandatory to determine if an abscess has formed which will need draining. A multi-disciplinary team is usually involved from maxillofacial surgery, ENT and ophthalmology.

Case 19

Candidates instruction:

You are the Foundation doctor on a GP placement. Your next patient is a 54 year old woman who has noticed the skin around her nose has changed and become red over the last few weeks. Take a short history and examine this patient presenting with nasal erythema.

After 6 minutes the examiner will stop you and ask you to summarise back your findings, suggest your management plan and answer some direct questions.

Examiner's instructions

This is a station where the candidate has to elicit a history of the presenting complaint. The candidate is then to perform a focused examination of a patient with facial erythema.

When the patient is being examined give the appropriate clinical findings if the candidate performs the correct examination technique or describes what they would like to do to elicit a clinical sign.

Ask the candidate to summarize their findings and offer a differential diagnosis with a management plan.

After 6 minutes, please stop the candidate and ask:

"Please summarise your findings and discuss how you would like to investigate and manage this patient."

Examination findings:

Observations
Comfortable at rest on room air
Respiratory rate 16, SpO2 100% on room air
Pulse 80, BP 150/95 Capillary refill time 3 seconds, Warm peripheries
36.5°

Inspection
Rash in a malar distribution
Nasolabial folds are spared

Palpation
Area not tender
Not warmth compared to other skin
Not raised

Actors instruction:

You are a 54 year old woman with a 2 week history of erythema around her nose.

You noticed a mild redness around your nose when you came back from holiday in Spain. You initially thought it was sunburn, but it has got worse and spread from your nose to your cheeks.

Your face feels quite puffy and sore.

You have been feeling quite run down and tired recently.

The rash itself is not tender

If directly asked, state that your joints have been hurting recently, especially in your hands.

You have no past medical history.

No regular medications. No known allergies. You take HRT for Menopause.

You live with your husband and 2 children. Smoke 10/day for the last 20 years and minimal alcohol. You are a housewife

No accurate family history, but you do remember a great aunt who always had a red face and was wheelchair bound before she died.

Your primary concern is that it may be cancer.

Case 19 Task:	Achieved	Not Achieved
Introduces self & clarifies who they are speaking to		
History:		
Specifically asks for: Onset of symptoms and relation to returning from holiday (sun exposure) Any tenderness across the rash Any associated joint pain		
Asks about any past medical, drug history & allergy and family history		
Examination:		
Checks bedside clinical observations		
Inspection/ Notes symmetrical appearance of rash Notes sparing of nasolabial folds		
Palpation/ Notes that area is not tender Notes area is not raised Examine regional lymph nodes (no lymphadenopathy elicited)		
Examination – Joints *If ascertained in history that has joint pain, offers to examine relevant joints (hands) – do not actually let candidate examine joints*		
Examination – examination of nose Offers to examine both nostrils		
Explores Ideas, concerns, and expectations		
Demonstrates good rapport and empathy with the patient		
Relays a concise summary to the examiner		
Offers differential diagnoses		
Management plan (3 marks) Complete examination by looking for other skin changes elsewhere and joint examination FNE to look for malignancy Blood tests for auto antibodies and renal function		
Examiner's Global Mark	/5	
Actor / Helper's Global Mark	/5	
Total Station Mark	/30	

Learning points:

- The patient has signs and symptoms suggestive of systemic lupus erythematosus (SLE). Other differentials include malignancy, sjogrens, sarcoidosis, dermatitis, sunburn, etc.

- Recognize that it is a systemic condition and offer to examine for joint involvement (hand examination).

- Recognize the need for further haemotological testing for auto antibodies, however can be a local reaction due to nasal pathology (malignancy), may require Fiber-optic Naso-endoscopy (FNE).

Case 20

Candidates instruction:

You are the Foundation doctor working at a GP practice. Your next patient complaints of noisy breathing and his nostrils feeling blocked. **Examine** this patient's nose

After 6 minutes the examiner will stop you and ask you to summarise back your findings, suggest your management plan and answer some direct questions.

Examiner's instructions:

When the patient is being examined give the appropriate clinical findings if the candidate performs the correct examination technique or describes what they would like to do to elicit a clinical sign.

Ask the candidate to summarize their findings and offer a differential diagnosis with a management plan.

After 6 minutes, please stop the candidate and ask:

"Please summarise your findings and discuss how you would like to investigate and manage this patient."

Examination findings:

There is no pain

There is no discharge

There is no erythema

Examination of the nose reveals a deviated septum towards the right with narrowing of the air passages.

Actors instruction:

You are a 46 year old man attending a GP practice. For years your partner has complained about your noisy breathing, especially at night. In addition to this you feel as if your right nostril is always blocked. As it has persisted you have come to the GP to find out what it is.

You are otherwise well.

Case 20 Task:	Achieved	Not Achieved
Introduces self and clarifies role		
Briefly explains examination and obtains consent		
Asks about any breathing problems		
Asks about pain		
Assessment of nose		
Assessment of external nose – skin changes, deviation of bones		
Checks airflow by isolating nostrils		
Uses Thudicums appropriately		
Selects appropriate light source		
Looks in all accessible regions of the non-symptomatic side first		
Checks for discharge		
Checks for masses / FB		
Repeats procedure on other nostril		
Identifies abnormality (septal deviation)		
Proceeds to check oropharynx		
States would then examine the ears		
Checks regional lymph nodes		
Offers to use a Fiber-optic Naso-endoscope to assess the nasopharynx/posterior nasal cavity		
Demonstrates good rapport with the patient throughout		
Relays a concise summary to the examiner		
Interprets findings adequately		
Examiner's Global Mark	/5	
Actor / Helper's Global Mark	/5	
Total Station Mark	/30	

Learning points:

- Air flow through both nostrils should be assessed first. Ask the patient to sequentially inhale and exhale sequentially through both nostrils. When examining the nasal cavity, open the nostrils using Thudicums (held using the thumb, fore and middle fingers). Ensure that you have an appropriate light source (either torch in other hand or headlamp) as you need to be able to visualize all areas of the nasal cavity

- One of the least invasive ways of examining the nasopharynx thoroughly in a clinic setting is by using a Fiber-optic Naso-endoscope

- As an examination of the nose/nasal cavity is incomplete without an oral exam, you should always offer to examine the oral cavity when faced with such a patient

Case 21

Candidates instruction:

You are the Foundation doctor working at a GP practice. Your next patient complains of a lump in her nose. **Examine** this patient presenting with a nasal lump

After 6 minutes the examiner will stop you and ask you to summarise back your findings, suggest your management plan and answer some direct questions.

Examiner's instructions:

When the patient is being examined give the appropriate clinical findings if the candidate performs the correct examination technique or describes what they would like to do to elicit a clinical sign.

Ask the candidate to summarize their findings and offer a differential diagnosis with a management plan.

After 6 minutes, please stop the candidate and ask:

"Please summarise your findings and discuss how you would like to investigate and manage this patient."

Examination findings:

There is no pain

There is no current discharge

Examination of the nose reveals an irregular raised lump on the inside of the left nostril fixed to skin and extending into the nasal cavity.

Actors instruction:

You are a 65 year old woman attending a GP practice. You have noticed this lump on the inside of your left nostril which has been growing over the last 3 months. It has bled intermittently. You are a lifelong smoker of 20/day but otherwise well. You are concerned it is cancer.

Case 21 Task:	Achieved	Not Achieved
Introduces self and clarifies role		
Briefly explains examination and obtains consent		
Asks about any breathing problems		
Assessment of nose		
Inspects for obvious nasal disfigurement		
Checks airflow by isolating nostrils		
Uses Thudicums and light source appropriately		
Assessment of nasal lump		
Assesses for erythema and warmth		
Assesses for a punctum or discharge		
Assesses if fixed to skin/underlying structures by placing the lump between 2 fingers and attempting to move it		
Assesses if compressible		
Assesses for overlying skin changes		
Repeats procedure on other nostril		
Identifies abnormality (lump fixed to skin)		
Proceeds to check oropharynx		
Offers to examine the ears		
Checks regional lymph nodes		
Offers to use a Fiber-optic Naso-endoscope to assess the nasopharynx/posterior nasal cavity		
Demonstrates good rapport with the patient throughout		
Relays a concise summary to the examiner		
Interprets findings adequately		
Examiner's Global Mark	/5	
Actor / Helper's Global Mark	/5	
Total Station Mark	/30	

Learning points:

- When examining an abnormality in part of the body organ with laterality, always (or offer to) start with the normal side first; in this case, the normal nostril first When inspecting the nasal cavity, open each nostril using the Thudicums held in thumb, middle and fore fingers. Offer to examine the oral cavity at the end of your exam, and also suggest using a Fiber-optic Naso-endoscope to assess the nasopharynx in more detail

- In this age group, it is important to rule out malignancy, and as such, this should be top of your differential list. Other differentials for a lump on the nose include a polyp, sebaceous cyst, a post-traumatic lesion, or other rheumatological/autoimmune lesions such as SLE, sarcoidosis etc.

- All lumps should be examined in a systematic manner in order to fully assess all aspects of the lump (size, shape, adherence to underlying structures including skin, overlying erythema/skin changes, compressibility, pulsatility, transluminence). In this case, remember to check the regional lymph nodes (in this case, around the neck and superior mediastinum)

Case 22

Candidate's instructions:

A 12-year old boy presents to the Emergency Department (ED) minor injuries unit with complications of nasal trauma he sustained recently. You are the Foundation year doctor in ED and you are asked by your consultant to take a short history from the patient and carry out the relevant clinical examination, and offer a management plan.

After 6 minutes the examiner will stop you and ask you to summarise back your findings, suggest your management plan and answer some direct questions.

Examiner's instructions:

This is a scenario of complicated nasal trauma in a 15 years old boy. The candidate is asked to take a history and carry out a comprehensive examination of the patient.

After 6 minutes, please stop the candidate and ask:

"Please summarise your findings and discuss how you would like to investigate and manage this patient."

Examination findings:

The physical examination should reveal:

1. An infected septum bilateral haematoma
2. A bony deformity of the nasal bones towards the left
3. No other neurological, orbital or maxillo-facial abnormalities
4. A temperature of 38.7 degrees
5. No neurological signs, your limbs and vision are normal
6. You have some mucky mucus in your nostrils but no blood and no watery discharge
7. The partition inside your nose is boggy and swollen filling your nostrils on both sides, and your nose skin is red and tender to touch
8. Your bony nose bridge is tender, mildly swollen and is deviated towards the left
9. You have no other facial deformities, bruising or tenderness

The candidate should suggest the following plan of action:

1. Admitting the patient and prepare him for a possible GA
2. Secure an IV access and take bloods for FBC, U&Es, CRP and clotting

3. Inform senior and discuss the need for IV antibiotics and for a manipulation of nasal bones and incision and drainage of nasal septum infected haematoma under GA
4. Counselling the patient and relatives regarding the diagnosis of nasal bones fracture and the need for manipulation under anaesthesia after 7-14 days from the trauma
5. Counselling patient and relatives regarding the diagnosis of an infected nasal septum haematoma and the need for an incision and drainage under GA to prevent the dissemination of sepsis

Actors instructions:

You are a 12-year old boy who has been fit and healthy previously. You have a healthy family, and have no allergies. You do not drink alcohol and do not smoke or take recreational drugs.

A week ago you were playing hide and seek with your parents and accidentally were head-butted during the game on your nose. You had instantly a nose bleed that stopped with pressure within a few minutes. You carried on playing and had no further problems that day, except for a mild swelling of your nose. The swelling progressed gradually then it had regressed over the last few days. However, the regression of the swelling has allowed you to notice that the bony part of your nose is squint towards the left hand side. Also, you have been troubled for few days with a worsening blockage of your nose.

Since yesterday, you have developed headaches all over your head and intermittent fevers but no vomiting, nausea or vision problems. Apart from the bleeding you had after the incident, you have had no further bleeding or any nasal discharge. You and your family are extremely concerned about your nose deformity and want it to be sorted so it does not affect your cosmetic appearance on a long term basis.

The candidate should be considerate, polite and professional.

He/she should introduce him/herself appropriately, explain what he/she intends to do, and wash his/her hands before and after the examination.

He/she should check what areas in your body are painful to be considerate towards these during the examination.

The candidate should ask you if you have any questions, and then should explain his/her findings and management plan to you and your family in lay terms.

Case 22 Task:	Achieved	Not Achieved
Introduces self & clarifies who they are speaking to		
Demonstrates an infection-control compliant approach: Bare below the elbow + washes hands at the start and at the end of the station		
Explains goal of encounter and seeks consent to proceed		
History:		
Takes a systematic pain history pain methodically (e.g. using "SOCRATES")		
Asks about time, date, and mechanism of injury		
Be specific and open regarding potential safeguarding issues (non-accidental injury, bullying etc.)		
Clarifies the onset and progress of nasal symptoms (bleeding, obstruction, anosmia, CSF leak)		
Asks about neurological and visual symptoms (headaches, nausea, diplopia etc)		
Ask about past and recent medical / surgical / medications history		
Checks social and family history		
Checks allergy status		
Examination:		
Checks (personally or ask for) basic observations: Temperature, HR, BP, SaO2 on air		
Considerately inspects and palpates the face for: Bleeding / bruising / deformity / tenderness / fractures		
Carries out nasal anterior examination for: Deformity / haematoma / bleeding / sniff test		
Carries out a brief neurological examination (cranial nerves, neck stiffness, pupils)		
Examine oral cavity for palate trauma / bleeding / teeth loosening		
Clarifies the patient's subjective feeling of facial deformity and explores the patient's and relatives' ideas, concerns, and expectations		

Demonstrates good rapport and empathy with the patient/relatives throughout		
Suggests a reasonable initial management plan		
Relays a concise summary of findings to the examiner		
Examiner's Global Mark	/5	
Actor / Helper's Global Mark	/5	
Total Station Mark	/30	

Learning points:

- Nasal deformities affect the central aesthetic compartment of the face, and are therefore markedly noted and well appreciated by the patients and their relatives. The concern is usually significant and can lead to psychological impact that should be approached considerately.

- The non-surgical management of nasal traumatic deformities is best achieved during the second week after the injury. During that period the swelling is usually regressed to allow precise appreciation of the bony deformity, and the fractured bones are still amenable to closed manipulation under GA.

- A nasal septum haematoma, if untreated, can commonly become infected and turn into a septum abscess. This can cause complicated nasal deformities which are difficult and complex to treat. More importantly, such sepsis can spread into the orbit, sinuses, meninges, and cavernous sinus. Therefore, the early recognition and prompt treatment of a nasal septum haematoma in nasal trauma are crucial.

Case 23

Candidate instructions:

You are the Foundation doctor in the ED and are asked to **examine** the nose of a 19-year-old male patient who presents with a bleeding nose after being assaulted outside a night club.

After 6 minutes the examiner will stop you and ask you to summarise back your findings, suggest your management plan and answer some direct questions.

Examiner's instructions:

This is a scenario of complicated nasal trauma in a 19 years old man. The candidate is asked to carry out a comprehensive examination of the patient's nose.

After 6 minutes, please stop the candidate and ask:

"Please summarise your findings and discuss how you would like to investigate and manage this patient."

Examination findings:

The bridge of the nose is deviated to the left and is tender.

There is a small laceration to the skin and a red eye.

No eye signs/andormailities.

There is obvious epistaixs, but no other nasal (CSF, catarhh etc) discharge.

Actor instructions:

You are a 19-year-old young male who was on a night out and was assaulted (ie: punched in the face) by two other guys. You just had a pint of beer and were not drunk. There was no other trauma and you feel fine and calm.

You don't think you lost much blood but it is still oozing slightly. You used a paper tissue to sustain the bleeding with good effect.

You did not lost consciousness and fully remember what happened. You do not have any other symptoms such as headaches or dizziness.

Case 23 Task:	Achieved	Not Achieved
Introduces self & clarifies who they are speaking to		
Washes hands		
Permission obtained to perform examination		
Exposes and re-positions the patient appropriately		
Briefly checks vital signs & evidence of significant blood loss		
Recognizes/looks for obvious external abnormalities such as: Trauma Bruising to the periorbital region/mastoid process Lacerations Symmetry/deviation of the nose Swelling to the face Tenderness of the facial bones on palpation		
Assess for nasal discharge and notes features such as : Bright red blood Volume Mucus/CSF		
Palpates: The nose for tenderness/obvious fractures The facial bones for tenderness/obvious fractures		
Appropriately inserts a nasal speculum		
Notes presence/absence of foreign objects		
Relays a concise summary to the examiner		
Mentions further assessments/tests required		
Examiner's Global Mark	/5	
Actor / Helper's Global Mark	/5	
Total Station Mark	/30	

Learning points:

- Epistaxis is commonly caused by trauma (including nose picking), iatrogenic (anticoagulants, surgery, cocaine), and bleeding disorders. The severity and onset of the haemorrhage define the most effective management (conservative, medical, or surgical). Therefore, thorough history taking is crucial in order to define the likely cause(s) and best management plan.

- Epistaxis patients are commonly under significant stress due to pain and anxiety. This usually causes tachycardia, a rise in blood pressure and subsequently a higher risk of bleeding. Therefore the patient's anxiety and pain must be promptly assessed and addressed, preferably through a methodical manner (e.g. SOCRATES).

- Although the cause can often be obvious such as in case of trauma, it is important to be methodical and look for cues and clues of other potential causes (eg: skin bruising can suggest anticoagulation use or coagulopathies)

Section 3

Throat & Head and Neck Cases

Case 24

Candidates instruction:

You are a Foundation doctor on a GP placement. Take a history from this 58 year old patient presenting with dysphagia.

After 6 minutes the examiner will stop you and ask you to summarise back your findings, suggest your management plan and answer some direct questions.

Examiner's instructions:

The station is directed towards history taking only and therefore the candidate should be reminded of that should they try to carry out a clinical examination.

After 6 minutes, please stop the candidate and ask:

"Please summarise your findings and discuss how you would like to investigate and manage this patient."

Actors instruction:

You are a 58 year old bricklayer attending GP with progressive difficulty in swallowing for the past 6 weeks. You previously ate a full normal diet but now find that solid food, such as meat, sticks in the throat and you have only been able to eat soup for the past 1 week. You can drink fluids although sometimes this causes you to cough and choke a little bit. Your appetite is reduced. Swallowing is not generally painful

You do not know exactly how much you weigh but your trousers are a little looser than last month. In the last week you have also noticed a small, firm, non-tender lump on the left side of your neck and pain in the left ear. No other ear symptoms. You have no difficulty in breathing and walked half a mile to the surgery today.

You take Amlodipine for high blood pressure and have no drug allergies. You have smoked 10-20 roll-up cigarettes every day since you were 17 years old and drink 2 pints of strong lager most evenings after work. You live with your wife of 35 years who thinks your voice is more hoarse than usual.

If asked, you are worried this might be a tumour as your father had throat cancer and died aged 55.

Case 24 Task:	Achieved	Not Achieved
Introduces self & clarifies who they are speaking to		
Specifically asks about: Onset of swallowing problem (gradual vs sudden) Difference between swallowing solids and liquids Associated pain Voice change Neck swellings Breathing difficulties Otalgia Halitosis Unintentional weight loss/Loss of appetite Night sweats General malaise/lethargy		
Asks about smoking/alcohol history and occupation		
Asks about past medical/surgical history		
Asks about Family history of malignancies		
Asks about drug history & compliance and allergy status		
Explores Ideas, concerns, and expectations		
Demonstrates good rapport and empathy with the patient throughout		
Relays a concise summary to the examiner		
Identifies the need to refer to secondary care via the 2 week wait suspected cancer pathway.		
Examiner's Global Mark	/5	
Actor / Helper's Global Mark	/5	
Total Station Mark	/30	

Learning points:

- Main differentials to exclude are:

  malignancy (malignant/benign), Zenker's diverticulum, GORD

- In any head and neck malignancy station, asking about weight loss, tolerance of solids/liquids, family history and a quantified smoking & alcohol history are key

- Remember to explore the non-malignancy differentials whilst taking a history. Singers are prone to having vocal cord polyps, and gastro-oesophageal reflux disease can also cause dysphagia

Case 25

Candidates instruction:

You are a Foundation doctor on a rotation at a GP practice. Take a comprehensive history from a 20-year old lady presenting with odynophagia

After 6 minutes the examiner will stop you and ask you to summarise back your findings, suggest your management plan and answer some direct questions.

Examiner's instructions:

The station is directed towards history taking only and therefore the candidate should be reminded of that should he/she try to carry out a clinical examination.

After 6 minutes, please stop the candidate and ask:

"Please summarise your findings and discuss how you would like to investigate and manage this patient."

Actors instruction:

You are a 20 year old student attending the GP practice with progressive difficulty in swallowing and worsening pain for the past 5 days, particularly on the right side.

You can feel large swellings under the jaw on both sides of your neck which are tender to palpate and have pain throbbing to the right ear. You have no ear discharge or loss of hearing. You have no difficulty in breathing but cannot open your mouth as wide as normal and your voice is altered ("Hot Potato voice"). In the last 24 hours you have been able to drink 1 litre of water but have not eaten since yesterday.

You have well controlled asthma and play Rugby 7s for your university. You have been taking regular Co-codamol from the pharmacy. You use a salbutamol inhaler regularly and avoid NSAIDS as they make you wheezy. Penicillin gives you a rash and swollen lips. You are a non-smoker and drink alcohol 1-2 times per week.

You are concerned that you are meant to be playing rugby at the weekend in an important Cup competition

Case 25 Task:	Achieved	Not Achieved
Introduces self & clarifies who they are speaking to		
Specifically asks about: Onset of swallowing problem (gradual vs sudden) Difference between swallowing solids and liquids Associated pain Voice change Neck swellings Breathing difficulties Otalgia Unintentional weight loss/loss of appetite Night sweats General malaise/lethargy		
Asks about smoking history and alcohol consumption		
Asks about past medical/surgical history		
Asks about Family history of malignancies		
Asks about drug history & compliance and allergy status		
Recent contact with someone with similar symptoms		
Explores Ideas, concerns, and expectations		
Demonstrates good rapport and empathy with the patient throughout		
Relays a concise summary to the examiner		
Identifies the likely underlying diagnosis of a peri-tonsillar abscess (quinsy)		
Examiner's Global Mark	/5	
Actor / Helper's Global Mark	/5	
Total Station Mark	/30	

Learning points:

- Main differentials to exclude are: acute tonsillitis, peri-tonsillar abscess, pharyngitis, malignancy

- In any head and neck malignancy station, asking about weight loss, tolerance of solids/liquids, family history and a quantifying smoking & alcohol history are key.

- Remember to explore the non-malignancy differentials whilst taking a history. Younger patients are less likely to have malignancy, so an infection should be higher up the differential list

Case 26

Candidates instruction:

You are a Foundation doctor on a rotation at a GP practice. Take a history from this 79-year old lady who presents with a lump in the throat

After 6 minutes the examiner will stop you and ask you to summarise back your findings, suggest your management plan and answer some direct questions.

Examiner's instructions:

The station is directed towards history taking only and therefore the candidate should be reminded of that should they try to carry out a clinical examination.

After 6 minutes, please stop the candidate and ask:

"Please summarise your findings and discuss how you would like to investigate and manage this patient."

Actors instruction:

You are a 79 year old retired Post Office worker attending the GP with a feeling of a lump in throat and progressive difficulty in swallowing over the past 5 months. Food seems to get stuck in the throat and occasionally you have to regurgitate it. You have noticed that occasionally you can feel a smooth soft swelling in the neck slightly to the left side. You were able to feel it this morning after a breakfast of tea and toast but it doesn't seem to be there now. Your husband complains that at times your breath smells and you get embarrassed by a gurgling sound that sometimes happens at meal times.

You have no pain on swallowing but have osteoarthritis affecting your neck and shoulders making it difficult to flex and extend your head. You have no difficulty breathing or talking although you have had 3 episodes of a chest infection in the last 6 months and had to be admitted to hospital for a pneumonia once.

You have well controlled hypertension and you take iron supplements. No allergies. You quit smoking 50 years ago and drink alcohol once per week at the most.

You are concerned that you have lost 5kg in the last 5 months and are worried you may have a cancer of the oesophagus.

Case 26 Task:	Achieved	Not Achieved
Introduces self & clarifies who they are speaking to		
Specifically asks about: Where is the 'lump in the throat' sensation felt		
Onset of symptoms		
Ability to swallow fluids and solids		
Associated pain		
Voice change		
Breathing difficulties		
Weight loss		
Recurrent chest infections		
Description of neck swelling: Position		
Size		
Shape – smooth/irregular		
Surface – hard/soft		
Asks about smoking history and alcohol consumption		
Asks about past medical/surgical history/drug history and allergy		
Explores Ideas, concerns, and expectations		
Demonstrates good rapport with the patient throughout		
Demonstrates empathy appropriately		
Relays a concise summary to the examiner		
Identifies the likely underlying diagnosis of a pharyngeal pouch		
Examiner's Global Mark	/5	
Actor / Helper's Global Mark	/5	
Total Station Mark	/30	

Learning points:

- A feeling of a 'lump in the throat' is a common presenting complaint but is vague and can mean different things to different people. The medical term for this is globus pharyngeus but it is essential that any significant pathology is not missed.

- This lady describes classical symptoms associated with a pharyngeal pouch (Zenker's diverticulum). Her lump is present when it fills with swallowed material. This can be confirmed with a barium contrast swallow and endoscopic stapling would be considered due to her recurrent aspiration pneumonia and weight loss.

- Differentials in this case: Pharyngeal pouch, extrinsic esophageal compression (e.g. cervical osteophyte), benign stricture (e.g. Plummer-Vinson syndrome), malignant stricture, neuromuscular oesophageal dysmotility.

Case 27

Candidates instruction:

You are a Foundation doctor on a rotation at a GP practice. Take a history from this 42-year old man who complains of tiredness and extreme day time somnolence.

After 6 minutes the examiner will stop you and ask you to summarise back your findings, suggest your management plan and answer some direct questions.

Examiner's instructions:

The station is directed towards history taking only and therefore the candidate should be reminded of that should he/she try to carry out a clinical examination.

After 6 minutes, please stop the candidate and ask:

"Please summarise your findings and discuss how you would like to investigate and manage this patient."

Actors instruction:

You are a 42 year old taxi driver attending the GP as you frequently feel tired at work and un-refreshed in the morning when you wake up. You go to bed at 11pm and wake several times in the night before rising to your alarm at 6am. Your wife complains that you snore very loudly. She occasionally makes you sleep in the spare room and she has taken a video of you sleeping where you hold your breath for 10-15 seconds before gasping and snoring loudly again. You often have a headache in the morning.

You smoke 15 cigarettes per day, drink alcohol 3 nights per week and you weigh 115kg. You are 5'9" (175cm) tall and your collar size is 18". You drink approx. 5 cups of coffee per day.

You have never been on any medication but recently had a blood test that showed a normal full blood count, renal function, thyroid function but your cholesterol is at the top of the normal range. You have some difficulty breathing through your nose since injuring it playing football 15 years ago so tend to sleep with your mouth open. You do not do any form of exercise presently.

You are concerned you may lose your job as you have started to take a nap in the afternoon and recently almost crashed into a parked car when you were feeling particularly tired. Your wife is concerned you might stop breathing altogether.

Case 27 Task:	Achieved	Not Achieved
Introduces self & clarifies who they are speaking to		
Specifically asks about: Normal bedtime and wake time routine		
Sleep fragmentation		
Sleep hygiene (i.e.: bedtime routine; presence of stimulation in sleeping environment such as noise, light)		
Do you snore		
Any reports of apnoea by family/friends		
Do you feel refreshed on waking		
Caffeine consumption		
Early morning headaches		
Smoking history		
Alcohol consumption		
Occupation history		
Any road traffic accidents or near misses		
Asks about past medical history		
Drug history and allergies		
Explores Ideas, concerns, and expectations		
Demonstrates good rapport with the patient throughout		
Demonstrates empathy appropriately		
Relays a concise summary to the examiner		
Directs the patient to inform the DVLA of likely OSA		
Examiner's Global Mark	/5	
Actor / Helper's Global Mark	/5	
Total Station Mark	/30	

Learning points:

- Obstructive sleep apnoea (OSA) is associated with being overweight, male, age >40 years, alcohol intake, smoking, sedative medication and family history. Poorly controlled OSA has a significant impact on quality of life and increases risk of cardiovascular events.

- Treatment options for OSA include lifestyle measures (e.g. weight loss, reduced alcohol and smoking cessation), Continuous Positive Airways Pressure (CPAP) to prevent airway collapse and oral appliances such as a Mandibular Advancement Device (MAD). Surgery to the nose, oropharynx or upper airway is considered in specific cases but should always be accompanied by applicable lifestyle measures.

- OSA can affect your ability to drive and it is the patient's legal responsibility to inform the Driver and Vehicle Licensing Agency (DVLA), hence why this patient's occupation is particularly relevant.

Case 28

Candidates instruction:

You are a Foundation doctor on a rotation at a GP practice. Take a **history** from this 29-year old who complains of voice hoarseness.

After 6 minutes the examiner will stop you and ask you to summarise back your findings, suggest your management plan and answer some direct questions.

Examiner's instructions:

The station is directed towards history taking only and therefore the candidate should be reminded of that should they try to carry out a clinical examination.

After 6 minutes, please stop the candidate and ask:

"Please summarise your findings and discuss how you would like to investigate and manage this patient."

Actors instruction:

You are a 29 year old drama teacher attending the GP as you have problem with your voice. You first noted this 3 months ago when you were producing and acting in a musical for 5 consecutive nights whilst feeling run down and suffering with a cold. It happened suddenly and you could not even perform on the last night when you lost your voice almost completely. You now find your voice quality gets more husky as the day goes on and when you teach evening classes you find it hard to project your voice adequately and the throat feels sore and strained.

Your voice is at its best first thing in the morning, although not perfect, and you noticed it was significantly better when you took 2 weeks off work for a relaxing holiday recently.

You smoke 5 cigarettes at the weekends, drink alcohol 2 nights per week. You drink approx. 1.5 litres of water a day and several cups of caffeinated tea. Your breathing is fine and you perform yoga twice a week.

You take the oral contraceptive pill and an over the counter vitamin supplement. You use a steroid inhaler for asthma. You have an allergy to latex, causing a rash. Alcohol and spicy foods give you gastric reflux. You have never had any surgery or a thyroid disorder.

You are concerned you may need surgery to your voice box and are nervous that your voice will never be the same again. You rely on your voice for work and you like to perform at open-mic nights but find your singing voice is very unreliable now.

Case 28 Task:	Achieved	Not Achieved
Introduces self		
Specifically asks about:		
Onset of symptoms – gradual/sudden		
Pattern of voice quality – fluctuating/constant		
Asks about voice use – work/recreation		
Asks about pain on phonation		
Enquires about difficulties breathing		
Enquires about difficulty swallowing		
Enquires about any neck lumps/swelling		
Enquires about indigestion/reflux		
Caffeine and water consumption		
Smoking history		
Alcohol consumption		
Occupation history		
Asks about past medical history		
Drug and allergy history		
Asks about previous surgery to the neck/mediastinum		
Explores Ideas, concerns, and expectations		
Demonstrates good rapport with the patient throughout		
Demonstrates empathy appropriately		
Relays a concise summary to the examiner		
Examiner's Global Mark	/5	
Actor / Helper's Global Mark	/5	
Total Station Mark	/30	

Learning points:

- Hoarseness or dysphonia are terms used to describe a change in voice quality. A thorough history must include details surrounding the onset of hoarseness, any change in voice quality through the day (reflux laryngitis is commonly worse in the morning, nodules worsen with voice use through the day), associated upper respiratory tract infection and voice use habits including occupation and leisure activities.

- A persistent hoarse voice for more than 2 weeks with no concurrent URTI in a patient over 45 years old meets criteria for a two week wait cancer pathway referral. Other red flags in the history include smoking, alcohol excess, a neck lump and associated stridor or dysphagia.

- In addition to benign and malignant vocal cord lesions it is important to consider pathology that may affect the innervation of the larynx via the superior laryngeal nerve or the recurrent laryngeal nerve.

Case 29

Candidates instruction:

You are the Foundation doctor in ENT, and have been asked to take a brief history and examine this 71-year old who presents with acute stridor

After 6 minutes the examiner will stop you and ask you to summarise back your findings, suggest your management plan and answer some direct questions.

Examiner's instructions

When the patient is being examined give the appropriate clinical findings if the candidate performs the correct examination technique or describes what they would like to do to elicit a clinical sign.

After 6 minutes, please stop the candidate and ask:

"Please summarise your findings and discuss how you would like to investigate and manage this patient."

Examination findings:

Patient appears panicked, sat upright and is using accessory muscles to breath

She can only give very short answers to questions, is in severe pain and is pointing to her neck

She appears in distress and is constantly spitting saliva into a bowl

A: Audible stridor from the foot of the bed

B: Appears peripherally cyanosed, but centrally well perfused

Respiratory rate is 40, Oxygen Sats on air 80%, on high flow oxygen 98%

Trachea is central, equal chest expansion and air entry bilaterally, chest percussion sounds normal >> no signs of a pneumothorax

C: Heart rate is 125 beats/minute, BP 170/88mmHg

D: She is fully alert but distressed

Actors instruction:

You are a 71 year retired secretary attending the emergency department with difficulty in breathing. This happened suddenly today at 1.30pm when you were eating in a restaurant with your family.

You finished your starter but whilst eating a rack of lamb your denture broke and you think you have swallowed either the denture or a piece of lamb bone. Since then you are making harsh rasping sound whenever you breath in and out.

You have pain at the level of your 'Adam's apple' which is worse when you try to talk or swallow. You are spitting out your saliva into a bowl.

You have previously had an anaphylactic allergy to shellfish and your daughter ate crab at the meal.

You are a non-smoker and drink in moderation. You had coronary artery bypass surgery 8 months ago and take Aspirin, Simvastatin, Clopidogrel and Ramipril.

Case 29 Task:	Achieved	Not Achieved
Introduces self & clarifies who they are speaking to		
History:		
Specifically asks about: Allergy		
Previous medical history/drug history/drug chart		
Timing/type of last meal/drink		
Events leading to presentation		
Enquires about difficulties breathing		
Enquires about difficulty swallowing		
Enquires about any neck lumps/swelling		
Assessment:		
Assesses airway – comments on stridor and applies Oxygen		
Palpate neck – site of pain and check trachea is central		
Checks for cyanosis		
Assess chest expansion		
Notes use of accessory muscles		
Auscultates chest		
Calculates respiratory rate accurately (within 2 breaths per minute)		
Attaches pulse oximeter or asks for 02 Sats		
Explores Ideas, concerns, and expectations		
Demonstrates good rapport with the patient throughout		
Demonstrates empathy appropriately		
Relays a concise summary to the examiner		
Examiner's Global Mark	/5	
Actor / Helper's Global Mark	/5	
Total Station Mark	/30	

Learning points:

- Stridor may be acute or chronic and can occur in childhood as well as adulthood. Stridor is distinct from stertor and may be inspiratory, expiratory or biphasic. Inspiratory stridor suggests a laryngeal obstruction, expiratory stridor suggests tracheobronchial obstruction and biphasic stridor suggests a glottic or subglottic obstruction.

- In an emergency, take an A.M.P.L.E. history and perform examination in a structured A.B.C. manner. With experience you will be able to do both these tasks simultaneously.

- AMPLE is primarily designed for trauma assessment but can be utilized in any emergent scenario where a concise history is required. AMPLE is Allergies, Medications, Previous medical/surgical history, Last meal time, Events surrounding injury/acute illness.

Case 30

Candidates instruction:

You are a Foundation doctor working in the emergency department. You have been asked to assess a 36 year man in the emergency department with difficulty in breathing. He has been brought in with significant facial injury following a motorbike accident. He now has increasing tongue swelling and is becoming drowsy.

Discuss the immediate and escalatory management of acute airway compromise.

You have 8 minutes for this station, but will get a warning bell 2 minutes prior to the end. Please use this remaining time to collect your thoughts and discuss any other important points you will like to cover.

Examiner's instruction:

At each stage press the candidate as to what the next step would be if that intervention failed. The patient suffered facial trauma and has a swollen tongue.

It is unknown whether he has a skull base fracture but he has no evidence of a cervical spine injury. He had morphine from the ambulance crew and has been given a dose of intravenous Co-Amoxiclav.

The tongue may be swollen due to haematoma or possibly allergic reaction to the antibiotic

The candidate has 8 minutes for this station, but please give them a warning with 2 minutes to go,

Patient Info:

36M, in ED resus. Trauma call patient; Motorbike versus lorry with significant facial injuries.

No known past medical, drug or allergy history.

He had morphine from the ambulance crew, and was been given a dose of intravenous Co-Amoxiclav on arrival in Resus.

Developed symptoms 15 minutes after the Co-Amoxiclav.

Initial assessment:
GCS E4 V2 M6
Tachypnoea (Resp rate 34)
Dyspnoea with increased drooling
Moderate bilateral air entry on auscultation

Patient appears well perfused, has a flushed sweaty face, and with distended neck veins + a swollen bloody protruding tongue

Further assessment:
GCS E2 V1 2   Resp rate 8
Reduced stridor   Minimal air entry bilaterally
Cyanosis involving the lips, reduced use of the accessory muscles, reduced chest movement
Nil change in neck swelling
Use of accessory respiratory muscles noted, with a marked effort of breathing

Case 30 Task:	Achieved	Not Achieved
Introduces self & clarifies who they are speaking to		
Identify airway compromise as an emergency situation, and refers to the ALS/ATLS guidelines		
Call for senior help (Cons/anesthetist/crash team)		
Applies high flow oxygen (15L/min) via non re-breathe mask		
Attach monitoring for oxygen saturations and pulse rate		
Consider treatment for anaphylaxis		
Considers any neck pathology **before** extending and manipulating the cervical spine		
Performs chin lift and head tilt		
Describes use of an oropharyngeal airway		
Able to choose correct size – corner of mouth to ear lobe		
Describes use of a nasopharyngeal airway		
Able to choose correct size – patient's little finger		
Aware of contraindications to NPA (i.e.: skull base fracture)		
Consider supraglottic airway device such as a laryngeal mask airway		
Describes endotracheal intubation		
Mentions video laryngoscopy to improve the view of the laryngeal inlet (e.g. GlideScope)		
Mentions need for rapid sequence induction		
Mentions option for awake fibreoptic nasal intubation		
Describes temporary surgical airway – crico-thyroidotomy		
Describes definitive surgical airway – surgical tracheostomy		
Examiner's Global Mark	/5	
Actor / Helper's Global Mark	/5	
Total Station Mark	/30	

Learning points:

- Airway compromise must be recognized as an emergency situation requiring senior assistance. Referring to guidelines such as ATLS is an excellent way to give your discussion structure.

- Consider whether there are any contraindications to your actions, especially in the context of trauma. Skull base fractures can make nasopharyngeal airway placement hazardous and cervical spine injuries may impact on the ability to manipulate the neck.

- A protected airway is defined as a cuffed tube inflated below the glottis. Although a supraglottic airway allows for positive pressure ventilation and obstructs the oesophagus it does not protect the airway from aspiration in the same way as a cuffed endotracheal tube. (ETT)

Case 31

Candidates instruction:

You are a Foundation doctor on a GP placement. Take a history from this 79 year old lady who presents with a lump in the throat

After 6 minutes the examiner will stop you and ask you to summarise back your findings, suggest your management plan and answer some direct questions.

Examiner's instructions:

The station is directed towards history taking only and therefore the candidate should be reminded of that should he/she try to carry out a clinical examination.

After 6 minutes, please stop the candidate and ask:

"Please summarise your findings and discuss how you would like to investigate and manage this patient."

Actors instruction:

You are a 79 year old retired Post Office worker attending the GP with a feeling of a lump in throat and progressive difficulty in swallowing over the past 5 months. Food seems to get stuck in the throat and occasionally you have to regurgitate it. You have noticed that occasionally you can feel a smooth soft swelling in the neck slightly to the left side. You were able to feel it this morning after a breakfast of tea and toast but it doesn't seem to be there now. Your husband complains that at times your breath smells and you get embarrassed by a gurgling sound that sometimes happens at meal times.

You have no pain on swallowing but have osteoarthritis affecting your neck and shoulders making it difficult to flex and extend your head. You have no difficulty breathing or talking although you have had 3 episodes of a chest infection in the last 6 months and had to be admitted to hospital for a pneumonia once.

You have well controlled hypertension and you take iron supplements. No allergies. You quit smoking 50 years ago and drink alcohol once per week at the most.

You are concerned that you have lost 5kg in the last 5 months and are worried you may have a cancer of the oesophagus.

Case 31 Task:	Achieved	Not Achieved
Introduces self & clarifies who they are speaking to		
Specifically asks about: Where is the lump in the throat sensation felt		
Onset of symptoms		
Ability to swallow fluids and solids		
Associated pain		
Voice change		
Breathing difficulties		
Weight loss		
Recurrent chest infections		
Description of neck swelling:		
Position		
Size		
Shape – smooth/irregular		
Surface – hard/soft		
Asks about smoking history and alcohol consumption		
Asks about past medical/surgical/drug history & allergy		
Explores Ideas, concerns, and expectations		
Demonstrates good rapport with the patient throughout		
Demonstrates empathy appropriately		
Relays a concise summary to the examiner		
Identifies the likely underlying diagnosis of a pharyngeal pouch		
Examiner's Global Mark	/5	
Actor / Helper's Global Mark	/5	
Total Station Mark	/30	

Learning points:

- A feeling of a 'lump in the throat' is a common presenting complaint but is vague and can mean different things to different people. The medical term for this is globus pharyngeus but it is essential that any significant pathology is not missed.

- This lady describes classical symptoms associated with a pharyngeal pouch (Zenker's diverticulum). Her lump is present when it fills with swallowed material. This can be confirmed with a barium contrast swallow and endoscopic stapling would be considered due to her recurrent aspiration pneumonia and weight loss.

- Differentials in this case: Pharyngeal pouch, extrinsic esophageal compression (e.g. cervical osteophyte), benign stricture (e.g. Plummer-Vinson syndrome), malignant stricture, neuromuscular oesophageal dysmotility.

Case 32

Candidate's instructions:

You are an ED Foundation doctor. A 22-year old woman anxiously attends the emergency department (ED) with sudden palpitations and a progressively growing neck lump. The patient called her GP yesterday to book an appointment because of her neck swelling that has been increasingly growing over the past month. However, tonight she started having palpitations, shortness of breath and lightheadedness. The ED Nurse Practitioner who triaged the patient documented the following vitals (BP 140/90, HR 115, temp 37.5, SaO2 96% on air). Take a full history from this patient

After 6 minutes the examiner will stop you and ask you to summarise back your findings, suggest your management plan and answer some direct questions.

Examiner's instructions:

This is a scenario of a 22 year old woman who attends the emergency department (ED) with sudden palpitations and a progressively growing neck mass. The patient's presentation suggests thyrotoxicosis with a thyroid goitre and atrial fibrillation; the candidate should be able to elicit that through the information he/she gathers from the patient.

The station is directed towards history taking only and therefore the candidate should be reminded of that should he/she try to carry out a clinical examination.

After 6 minutes, please stop the candidate and ask:

"Please summarise your findings and discuss how you would like to investigate and manage this patient."

Actors instructions:

You are a 22 year old woman who attends the emergency department (ED) with sudden palpitations and a progressively growing neck swelling.

You have noticed in the middle of your neck a swelling that has been gradually growing over the past four weeks. The swelling is not tender and does not affect your voice, swallowing or breathing. Over the past month you have been troubled with many symptoms that are increasing in number and in severity. You have been troubled with marked irritability, sweating of palms and feet, and trembling of your hands. Despite having an excellent appetite, you have lost over half a stone in weight over the past month. Your periods have not changed, however your relationship with your boyfriend is strained due to your bad temper.

You have booked an appointment next week with your GP due to the neck swelling, and an appointment with the opticians as you have been getting blurring and double vision over the past two weeks.

Tonight, you woke up with a sudden feeling of palpitations that you thought were due to you being anxious. However, your palpitations persisted for longer than an hour, so you attend ED. You have tremor in your hands and are feeling very anxious, short of breath and light-headed.

You have not had trauma, foreign travel, or illnesses recently. Your medical history includes resolved childhood asthma and an appendicectomy at the age of 13. The only medicine you take is the oral contraceptive pill; you are allergic to latex.

You work as a freelance artist, smoke only marijuana occasionally, and drink 30 units weekly of alcohol. Your mother has systemic lupus erythematosus and you lost your father to a heart attack.

The candidate will take a history from you about your symptoms in 7 minutes. Remember that you are very anxious, shaky-handed and short-tempered.

Case 32 Task:	Achieved	Not Achieved
Introduces self		
Explains goal of encounter and consent to proceed		
Asks if the patient wants a chaperone		
Clarifies if the patient has (and expresses willingness to address) any pain, discomfort, or needs methodically (e.g. "SOCRATES")		
Specifically asks about the following (one point each): The history of neck lump (onset, change in size, aggravating / relieving factors) Preceding events (trauma, travel, surgery, dental) Local symptoms (pain, tenderness, skin changes) Head and neck symptoms (dysphonia, dysphagia, odynophagia, sore throat, otalgia) Cardio-respiratory symptoms (chest pain, SOB, palpitations, cough, wheeze) General symptoms (weight, appetite, fevers) MSK symptoms: weakness in upper arms/thighs Neurological symptoms (headaches, vision, mood, dizziness) GU symptoms (urinary, periods, and ALWAYS LMP)		
Checks social / family history		
Checks past and recent medical / surgical history		
Checks drug history and allergy		
Elicits history in a concise and clear manner		
Explores the patient's and relative's ideas, concerns, and expectations		
Demonstrates good rapport and empathy with the patient and relatives throughout the encounter		
Relays a concise summary to the examiner		
Examiner's Global Mark	/5	
Actor / Helper's Global Mark	/5	
Total Station Mark	/30	

Learning points:

- The differential diagnosis of a neck lump covers a wide range of conditions that can be classified into congenital, inflammatory, endocrine, and neoplastic. The associated systemic and local involvement can be significant, such as AF and extensive anxiety in this case. Therefore, a comprehensive history taking is crucial to identify the likely diagnoses and initiate a plan of action.

- The systemic effects of endocrine neck masses can lead to significant cardiovascular and neurological duress. The patient's anxiety and pain must be promptly assessed and addressed, preferably through a methodical approach (e.g. SOCRATES).

- A calm, confident, and reassuring approach by the doctor can play a key role in addressing the patient's anxiety. Good rapport with the patient and relatives also assists the doctor in establishing a clear coherent history and gaining the patient's trust (reflected here in higher points rewarded).

Case 33

Candidate's instructions:

You are the Foundation doctor in ENT outpatients and you are sitting in the head and neck consultant-led clinic. You are asked by your consultant to carry out a clinical examination of a 45 years old male patient who has a history of a progressively enlarging, but otherwise asymptomatic, right sided neck lump.

After 6 minutes the examiner will stop you and ask you to summarise back your findings, suggest your management plan and answer some direct questions.

Examiner's instructions:

The candidate is tasked to carry out a comprehensive clinical examination of a 45 years old man who presents to the head and neck clinic with a right sided neck mass that has been gradually enlarging over two months. The patient is concerned that this mass is malignant due to a family history of cancer.

The session is aimed towards a clinical examination only, and the candidate should be reminded of that should he/she attempt to take any history.

After 6 minutes, please stop the candidate and ask:

"Please summarise your findings and discuss how you would like to investigate and manage this patient."

After summarising their findings, the candidate should conclude that the patient requires an urgent workup of the potentially neoplastic presentation. Within the outpatient setting the candidate should request (or perform if capable) an FNE, and a fine needle aspiration for cytology of the mass (FNAC).

The most prudent first line investigations of the neck node should include imaging (MRI neck) and blood testing (blood film, FBC, LFT's, U&Es, LDH, Viral serology [EBV/CMV/HIV], other serology [Bartonella / Toxoplasmosis], ESR / CRP, autoimmune profile [ANCA / RF]). Pending the results, second line investigations could include further imaging studies (USS / CT), TB testing, and a pan-endoscopy +/- node biopsy under GA.

Examination findings:

The examination reveals no upper airway noises and a normal.

The patient is well hydrated, has a normal weight, and his basic observations are (temperature 36.3, BP 140/85, HR 90, RR 14, SaO2 97% on air).

The inspection and palpation of the neck reveal a 5X5cm right sided firm neck mass at the upper half of the sternocleidomastoid muscle (levels 2&3). The lump is mobile, non-tender, not associated with skin changes and does not move on swallowing.

The examination of the oral cavity and oropharynx shows no abnormalities.

Facial inspection and anterior nasal examinations are unremarkable, and the patient has no other palpable masses.

If fibre-optic Naso-endoscopy (FNE) is available (even if only by an illustration that is provided to the candidate), it will be normal.

Actors instructions:

You are a 45 years old man who is being seen at the ENT clinic for a lump that has been gradually growing over the past two months in the right side of your neck. Apart from the lump you feel otherwise well in yourself and have had no issues with your breathing, voice, swallowing or weight. You have a firm non-tender swelling on the right hand side of your neck that doesn't move with your swallowing. Your examination will otherwise reveal no abnormalities.

You are very worried that the lump is cancerous as you lost your father to an oesophageal cancer 2 years ago.

The candidate should be considerate, polite and professional. They should introduce themselves appropriately, explain what they intends to do, and wash his/her hands before and after the examination. They should check what areas in your body are painful to be considerate towards these during the examination. The candidate should ask you if you have any questions or concerns, and then should explain their findings and management plan to you in lay terms and in a considerate manner towards your anxiety.

Case 33 Task:	Achieved	Not Achieved
Introduces self & clarifies who they are speaking to		
Explains the goal of the encounter and acquires consent to proceed		
Asks the patient for any painful / tender areas to be considerate towards these during examination		
Demonstrates an infection-control compliant approach		
Assesses for upper airway noises (stridor, stertor, gurgling, normal)		
Checks the patient's basic observations (temperature, BP, HR, RR, SaO2 on air)		
Carries out a general assessment of the patient (BMI, skin turgor, nail changes, peripheral oedema, bruising)		
Assesses the patient's voice quality (hoarse / breathy / strained / normal)		
Carries out a full inspection of the neck lump commenting on: scars, colour, symmetry or sinus		
Attempts to transilluminate the neck lump		
Carries out palpation of all neck regions (all 5 levels of the neck, thyroid gland, sub-clavicular, supra-clavicular, peri-auricular, TMJ's, occipital, and parotids), and systematically describes palpable masses (location, size, texture, mobility, tenderness, mobility)		
Carries out full oral cavity inspection (floor of mouth, buccal vestibules, gums, retro-molar areas, hard and soft palate, and oropharynx)		
Carries out a bimanual palpation of the floor of mouth (masses, stones), and massages the parotids while inspecting the parotid drainage points (opposite to upper second molars)		
Examines (or expresses will to) other lymph node regions (axillary, inguinal, popliteal)		
Demonstrates good rapport and empathy with the patient and relatives throughout the encounter		

Explains considerately and in lay-terms the examination findings and the needed further management steps to the patient and relatives		
Relays a concise summary of findings to the examiner		
Lists further clinical examinations that are required (FNE, FNAC)		
Lists required blood tests (blood film, FBC, LFT's, U&Es, LDH, infections serology, inflammatory markers, auto-antibodies)		
Suggests required imaging (USS / MRI / CT)		
Examiner's Global Mark	/5	
Actor / Helper's Global Mark	/5	
Total Station Mark	/30	

Learning points:

- A neck node in an adult should be assessed comprehensively to rule out neoplasia. A full ENT and head and neck assessment is vital in order to exclude / diagnose a primary site of the suspected malignancy.

- Vital diagnostic tests are available in outpatient settings (FNAC, FNE) and should be performed / requested to assist the diagnosis making process.

- Patients who present with neck masses are commonly concerned regarding a possible malignancy. Clinicians should follow a professional and considerate approach in order to facilitate the clinical examination, gain trust and build rapport with the patient and his/her relatives.

Case 34

Candidate's instructions:

You are a Foundation doctor sitting in the thyroid consultant-led clinic in ENT outpatients. You are asked by your consultant to carry out a clinical examination of the thyroid status of a 22-year old anxious woman who is referred by her GP with an enlargement of her thyroid gland.

The station should take 8 minutes in total, with a warning bell 2 minutes prior to the end, and the last 1 minute for a clear summary and presentation of the examination findings, differentials and to suggest a further management plan.

You are not required to carry out any history taking. You might use the provided pen and paper to take notes as required.

Examiner's instructions:

The candidate is tasked to carry out a comprehensive clinical examination of the thyroid status of a 22- year old woman who presents to the ENT thyroid clinic with an enlarging thyroid gland. The patient is very anxious, hyperventilating and complains of palpitations.

After 6 minutes, please stop the candidate and ask:

"Please summarise your findings and discuss how you would like to investigate and manage this patient."

After summarising their findings, the candidate should conclude that the diagnosis is that of a thyrotoxic thyroid goitre and atrial fibrillation. There is a possible retrosternal extension but no airway compromise. The candidate should recommend an urgent workup of the patient's cardiac status through an ECG, blood testing (U&Es, Ca, Mg) and a medical / cardiology referral. From a thyroid point of view, the candidate should propose a FNE to assess the vocal cords, an ultrasound scan (USS) guided fine needle aspiration of the thyroid mass (FNAC), and blood tests (FBC, TSH, T4/T3, thyroid auto-antibodies).

Examination findings:
The clinical examination of the patient reveals warm sweaty hands with fine tremor.

The patient has otherwise a normal examination of her skin, hair, muscular tone, and tendon reflexes.

She has mild upper eyelid retraction and a mild proptosis but otherwise a normal eye examination.

There is observable anxiety, with an irregularly irregular pulse; the observations read as HR 115, PB 140/90, RR 20, on air SaO2 100%, and temperature 37.

There are no upper airway noises, the voice is normal and her cough is strong.

The neck inspection shows a central symmetrical enlargement in the thyroid gland area with no skin changes otherwise.

Palpating the neck should reveal a symmetrical, non-tender, warm and smooth thyroid mass that moves on swallowing but not on tongue protrusion; no other masses are palpable.

There is no thyroid or carotid bruit but the percussion over the sternum manubrium is slightly dull.

Actors instructions:

You are a 22-year old woman who is being seen at the ENT clinic for a gradually enlarging thyroid gland over the past few weeks. During the consultation, you are very anxious, hyperventilating and are having palpitations in your chest. You have warm sweaty hands that have been trembling for few weeks. You have no problems with your skin, hair, muscles or limbs, but your eyes are protruding more and your eyelids are more open than usual. You have an irregular pulse but you have a normal voice, breathing and cough. Your neck is showing an obvious central enlargement of your thyroid gland but there are no other visible changes of the skin of your neck.

When the candidate feels your neck, they will be able to appreciate a thyroid enlargement that is symmetrical, non-tender, warm, smooth, and moves on swallowing but not on tongue protrusion. You have no other palpable lumps and the auscultation of your neck is normal. The percussion over the top part of your chest is slightly dull.

They should introduce him/herself appropriately, explain what they intends to do, and wash his/her hands before and after the examination. They should check what areas in your body are painful to be considerate towards these during the examination. The candidate should ask you if you have any questions or concerns, and then should explain their findings and management plan to you in lay terms. It is important that the candidate shows ability to deal with your anxiety appropriately and reassuringly, especially when he/she tells you that you have an irregular pulse that requires urgent investigations and an expert opinion.

Case 34 Task:	Achieved	Not Achieved
Introduces self		
Explains objectives and obtain consent to proceed		
Asks the patient for any painful / tender areas to be considerate towards these during examination		
Demonstrates an infection-control compliant approach		
Assesses the patient's hands (warmth / sweating / tremor), skin (dry / rough / thinning / oedema), and hair (thinning / hair loss)		
Checks the patient's muscles (stiffness / wasting) and tendon reflexes (delayed, hyper-reflexic)		
Assesses the patient's eyes for proptosis / lid lag / chemosis / reduced acuity		
Assesses the patient's pulse (regularity / rate), BP, weight, anxiety, temperature, RR, SaO2 on air		
Assesses for upper airway noises (stridor, stertor, gurgling, normal)		
Assesses the quality of the patient's voice (hoarse / breathy / strained / normal) and cough (strong / weak)		
Inspects the neck in a slightly forward flexed position at rest, and comment on any masses / scars / colour / symmetry / sinus		
Inspects the neck in a slightly forward flexed position during swallowing, and comment on any masses / scars / colour / symmetry / sinus		
Palpates the thyroid mass standing behind the patient and describes its symmetry / nodularity / movement with swallowing / movement with tongue protrusion / tenderness / warmth / size / laterality / consistency		
Auscultates for bruits over the thyroid and carotids		
Percusses over the sternum to rule out a retro-sternal extension of the thyroid mass		
Palpates all other neck regions to describe any other masses in a similar systematic method		

Demonstrates good rapport and empathy throughout the encounter, and explains in lay-terms the examination findings and the needed further management steps		
Relays a concise summary of findings to the examiner		
Recognises AF and recommends urgent tests (ECG, U&Es, Ca, Mg) and an urgent medical / cardiology opinion		
Recommends FNE, USS + FNAC and blood tests (FBC, TSH, T4/T3, thyroid antibodies) +/- MRI neck		
Examiner's Global Mark	/5	
Actor / Helper's Global Mark	/5	
Total Station Mark	/30	

Learning points:

- The initial presentation of thyroid diseases can be associated with systemic complications. Therefore, the assessment should be broad and inclusive of all systems that might be involved in the pathophysiology.

- A patient with a thyrotoxic neck lump presents commonly with significant distress that is related to their anxiety over the diagnosis and to the added significant systemic duress. Therefore, the patient anxiety and pain must be promptly and considerately addressed. A calm, confident, and reassuring approach by the doctor can play a key role in addressing the patient's anxiety.

- The cardiac manifestations of thyroid diseases can present acutely. Such presentations could lead to life threatening complications (Acute cardiac failure, arrhythmias, embolic events, thyroid storm). Therefore, suspected systemic acute complications should be addressed promptly and systematically, and should warrant an urgent referral for a medical expert opinion.

Case 35

Candidate's instructions:

You are the Foundation doctor in ENT; you are asked by your consultant to carry out a clinical examination of a patient who is being admitted to the ward from clinic. The patient is a 65 years old man with a history of increasing dysphonia (hoarseness) and dysphagia for few weeks.

After 6 minutes the examiner will stop you and ask you to summarise back your findings, suggest your management plan and answer some direct questions.

Examiner's instructions:

The candidate's task is to carry out a comprehensive clinical examination of a 65 years old man who presented with a few weeks history of dysphonia and dysphagia.

The session is aimed towards a clinical examination only, and the candidate should be reminded of that should they attempt to take any history.

After 6 minutes, please stop the candidate and ask:

"Please summarise your findings and discuss how you would like to investigate and manage this patient."

The candidate should summarise their findings as above and conclude the following points:

1. The patient is likely to be suffering with aspiration pneumonia and malnutrition because of dysphagia and aspiration
2. The patient has a likely thyroid mass that is causing the dysphonia (recurrent laryngeal nerve), dysphagia (invasion, external pressure) and aspiration (secondary to dysphagia, superior laryngeal nerve invasion)
3. The patient requires an urgent FNE
4. The required investigations are (FBC, U&Es, LFT's, Mg, PO4, TFT's, CXR, barium swallow, MRI neck +/- CT thorax)
5. The candidate should conclude the need to treat the aspiration pneumonia and to pass an NG tube for feeding

Examination findings:

The patient has the following examination findings:

1. No upper airway noises
2. Observations: apyrexial, BP 110/50, HR 105, RR 24, SaO2 92% on air)
3. BMI of 19, poor skin turgor, and mild peripheral oedema
4. A hoarse voice
5. The patients' neck inspection reveals a para-median thyroid area swelling on the right side with no skin other visual changes
6. The palpation reveals a firm right sided 4cm by 4cm thyroid mass that is multi-nodular, non-tender, fixed to deep structures and moves with swallowing
7. Normal oral cavity and oropharynx
8. Normal cranial nerve examination
9. Right base chest crepitations and dullness on percussion

Actors instructions:

You are a 65 years old man who is being admitted from clinic to the ENT ward as you have been suffering with a difficult swallowing and a hoarse voice for few weeks.

You have a slightly raised heart rate, poor skin elasticity and retention of fluids in your extremities because of your malnourishment. Also you have signs of a chest infection which is the result of your poor swallowing and aspiration. Your breathing is not noisy but you have a firm non-tender neck swelling on the right hand side that moves with your swallowing. Otherwise, your examination is unremarkable.

They should introduce themselves appropriately, explain what they intends to do, and wash their hands before and after the examination. They should check what areas in your body are painful to be considerate towards these during the examination. The candidate should ask you if you have any questions, and then should explain their findings and management plan to you in lay terms.

Case 35 Task:	Achieved	Not Achieved
Introduces self & clarifies who they are speaking to		
Explains goal of encounter and consent to proceed		
Asks the patient for any painful / tender areas to be considerate towards these during examination		
Checks for drug allergies		
Demonstrates an infection-control compliant approach		
Assesses for upper airway noises: (Stridor, stertor, gurgling, normal)		
Checks (personally or asks for) the patient's basic observations (temperature, BP, HR, RR, SaO2 on air)		
Carries out a general assessment of the nutritional state of the patient who presents with dysphagia: BMI, skin turgor, nail changes, peripheral oedema		
Assesses the patient's voice quality: Hoarse, breathy, strained, normal		
Neck inspection - Carries out an inspection of: Skin (scars, colour, symmetry, sinus) Masses (location, size, texture, mobility, tenderness, mobility)		
Carries out a neck palpation for masses / nodes including all 5 neck levels, thyroid, sub-clavicular area, supra-clavicular area, peri-auricular, TMJ, occipital area, and parotid		
Inspections of oral cavity (floor of mouth, buccal vestibules, gums, retro-molar areas, hard and soft palate, and oropharynx)		
Carries out a full cranial nerve examination		
Carries out or expresses need to do a chest examination (auscultation, percussion) to rule out aspiration		
Demonstrates good rapport and empathy with the patient and relatives throughout the encounter		
Explains in lay-terms the examination findings and the needed further steps of diagnosis to the patient		
Relays a concise summary of findings to the examiner		

Lists further clinical examinations that are required (FNE)		
Lists required laboratory tests (FBC, U&Es, LFT's, Mg, PO4, TFT's)		
Lists required radiological tests (Barium swallow, Video fluoroscopy, CT Thorax, MRI neck)		
Examiner's Global Mark	/5	
Actor / Helper's Global Mark	/5	
Total Station Mark	/30	

Learning points:

- A wide range of conditions can cause dysphagia and / or dysphonia. The clinician should bear in mind neurological, head and neck, thoracic and GI causes. A comprehensive clinical assessment is vital in order to recognise the likely cause and identify the best management plan.

- The causative pathology and consequences of dysphagia / dysphonia can compromise the patient's airway, nutritional status, and other systems (respiratory complications in this case). Therefore, the clinician should assess simultaneously the patient for any possible complications, particularly the airway.

- The clinician should follow a professional considerate approach towards the patient in order to facilitate the clinical examination, gain their trust and build rapport with the patient and relatives.

Case 36

Candidate's instructions:

You are the Foundation doctor in the ENT outpatient clinic. You are assessing a 35 year- old male patient who was referred urgently by their GP with a bleeding oral lesion. You have established from your history taking that the patient is fit and healthy, is a non-smoker, and drinks alcohol socially. The patient has been troubled for many years with a previously asymptomatic warty lesion on the oral aspect of his left cheek. However, the lesion that remains painless has enlarged and started bleeding over the past 4 weeks. The patient remains well and describes no symptoms otherwise. He has an unremarkable dental history, no dentures, and undergoes regular dentist checks twice yearly. PLease **Examine** this patient's mouth.

After 6 minutes the examiner will stop you and ask you to summarise back your findings, suggest your management plan and answer some direct questions.

Examiner's instructions:

The candidate is required to carry out a comprehensive clinical examination of a 35 years old man who presents with a bleeding lesion of his oral cavity. The history and examination should, overall, point towards a papilloma like lesion that is suspected to undergo a neoplastic change.

The OSCE is aimed towards a clinical examination only, and the candidate should be reminded of that should they attempt to take any history.

After 6 minutes, please stop the candidate and ask:

"Please summarise your findings and discuss how you would like to investigate and manage this patient."

Examination findings:

A 1X1cm left side warty / papillomatous buccal mucosa lesion that is ulcerated, covered with spots of clotted blood, non-tender, and positioned about 2cm anterior to the left palatine tonsil.
A healthy buccal mucosa otherwise
A left sided non-tender 2X2cm level III neck mass that is mobile underneath the skin and over deeper structures, doesn't move with swallowing, and is not associated with any skin changes
Normal weight, observations, and general assessment
Normal mouth opening, neck movements, voice, and airway noises
Normal lips, teeth, gums, and tongue assessment
Satisfactory examination of the floor of mouth, and oropharynx.

The candidate should summarise that this patient has a suspicious left sided oral lesion with an ipsilateral neck node. The candidate should recommend an urgent biopsy under LA or GA and an urgent MRI scan of the neck.

Actors instructions:

You are a 35 year-old man who is being seen urgently at the ENT outpatient clinic. You have had a warty lesion on the inside of your left cheek for many years. Recently, you have noticed that this lesion is changing in appearance, growing in size and bleeding intermittently. You have no pain or any other symptoms, and you have been fit and well previously. You are not sure why the lesion has become problematic and are concerned as to what the diagnosis might be.

The candidate is assessing you and is tasked to carry out an examination of your oral cavity and a relevant general examination. They should introduce themselves appropriately, explain what they intends to do, and wash their hands before and after the examination. They should check what areas in your body are painful to be considerate towards these during the examination. The candidate should ask you if you have any questions or concerns, and then should explain their findings and management plan to you in lay terms and in a considerate manner.

Your examination will show the following findings:

A 1X1cm left side warty lesion on the inside lining of your cheek that is ulcerated, covered with spots of clotted blood, and is non tender

A left sided neck lump that is 2X2 cm in dimensions, non-tender, mobile underneath the skin and over deeper structures, doesn't move with swallowing, and is not associated with any skin changes

A healthy examination of your mouth, throat and neck otherwise
Normal weight, observations, and general assessment

Case 36 Task:	Achieved	Not Achieved
Introduces self & clarifies who they are speaking to		
Explains the goal of the encounter and acquires consent to proceed		
Asks the patient for any painful / tender areas to be considerate towards these during examination		
Demonstrates an infection-control compliant approach		
Assesses mouth opening to rule out trismus and neck movements for torticollis		
Assesses lips (skin and mucosa) for any discolorations, lesions, or swellings		
Assesses teeth (decay, discoloration, malocclusion, dentures) and gums (lesions, discoloration, swelling, general health)		
Assesses with two tongue depressors (one inside each cheek for comparison) the buccal mucosa for discolorations, lesions, swellings, and excretion of saliva from parotid gland ducts		
Assesses the tongue: inspection (lesions / swellings / discolorations), movements (anterior and side to side protrusions / elevation), and palpation (submucosal lesions)		
Assesses the floor of mouth: inspection (lesions / swellings / discoloration / submandibular gland excretion), and bimanual palpation (through the neck and floor of the mouth for masses, tenderness or stones)		
Depresses the tongue in the midline with a tongue depressor to assess the palate, uvula, palatine tonsils, and oropharynx		
Assesses for upper airway noises (stridor, stertor, gurgling, normal) and checks the patient's basic observations (temperature, BP, HR, RR, SaO2 on air)		
Carries out a general assessment of the patient (BMI, skin turgor, nail changes, peripheral oedema)		
Assesses the patient's voice quality (hoarse / breathy / strained / normal)		
Carries out a full assessment of the neck including an inspection (scars, skin, sinus, lumps) and a palpation		

Demonstrates good rapport and empathy with the patient and relatives throughout the encounter		
Explains considerately and in lay-terms the examination findings and the needed further management steps to the patient and relatives		
Relays a concise summary of findings to the examiner		
Suggests a review of the patient's bedside observations, a thorough ENT history to include their past medical and family history, and a full ENT examination		
Suggests an urgent MRI of the neck, and an urgent excision biopsy (GA or LA) of the buccal lesion		
Examiner's Global Mark	/5	
Actor / Helper's Global Mark	/5	
Total Station Mark	/30	

Learning points:

- Oral pathologies should be thoroughly assessed to exclude malignancies. The lack of smoking history and the younger age of the patient should not rule out a neoplastic pathology; Human Papilloma Virus (HPV) related oral cancer can happen in non-smoking younger adults.

- A comprehensive oral, head & neck and general examination is crucial in order to evaluate the patient's lesion, and any spread in case of a suspected cancer. Please note that a comprehensive examination of the neck should include palpation of the lymph nodes in all '5 levels of the neck'; lymph nodes to in the submandibular, sub-clavicular, supra-clavicular, peri-auricular and occipital regions, and the temporo-mandibular joints (TMJs), thyroid gland, and parotid glands

- Patients who present with enlarging bleeding lesions are commonly concerned regarding a possible malignancy. Clinicians should follow a professional and considerate approach in order to facilitate the clinical examination, gain trust and build rapport with the patient and his/her relatives.

Case 37

Candidate's instructions:

You are the Foundation doctor in the ENT outpatient clinic. You are assessing a 35 year old woman who was referred by their GP via the choose and book system with left sided cheek tenderness and difficulties eating. Please **Examine** this patient's salivary glands

After 6 minutes the examiner will stop you and ask you to summarise back your findings, suggest your management plan and answer some direct questions.

Examiner's instructions:

The candidate is required to carry out a comprehensive clinical examination of a 35 year old woman who presents with bilateral parotid glands swelling, associated left sided gland tenderness and reduced salivation making eating difficult.

This patient presents with a clinical picture of Sjögren's syndrome, and the candidate is expected to recognize this, and tailor the exam in such a fashion.

The candidate should summarise that this patient has bilateral diffuse swellings of the parotid glands, a tender left parotid gland with associated expression of pus on palpation of the left gland. These findings in conjunction with the generalized sicca symptoms suggest a diagnosis of Sjögren's syndrome with a left sided infective parotitis.

The session is aimed towards a clinical examination only, and the candidate should be reminded of that should he/she attempt to take any history.

After 6 minutes, please stop the candidate and ask:

"Please summarise your findings and discuss how you would like to investigate and manage this patient."

Examination findings:

Besides a temperature of 38.1°C, the patient had normal bedside clinical observations
Normal sub-lingual/mandibular gland examinations (nil tenderness or swelling on palpation)

Bilateral diffuse parotid swellings

Left sided gland (parotid) tenderness

Nil overlying skin changes, nil temperature. The parotid swellings are soft, heterogeneous, and are not adherent to underlying structures.

When the glands are milked, there is an offensive thick yellow discharge from the left Stensen's (parotid) duct. Nothing was produced in the right parotid, or any of the other glands.

On inspection of the oral cavity, there were dried crusted food debris in the mouth, halitosis, ulcers over the tip of the tongue and obvious xerostomia

The patient was generally dry with minimal sweat production, had keratoconjuctivitis sicca (dry + red inflamed eyes), and dental caries

There was Left sided cervical (non-tender) lymphadenopathy

Actors instructions:

You are a previously fit and well 35 year old woman referred by your GP because you have complained of a 3 month history of bilateral cheek swellings, and have recently (4 day history) developed a left sided cheek tenderness, worse on eating and when you touch it. You have also been shaking and rigoring with a high temperature since this pain started, and can feel some non-tender rubbery lumps on the left side of your neck.

Something else you have noticed is that you're now having to chew a lot of 'minty' gums as your mouth gets dry easily, often smells 'rather awful' and have been producing thick offensive yellowish saliva, mostly from the left side of your mouth.

Eating has been difficult recently because of the mouth dryness. Your eyes are also increasingly red, itchy and dry, you sweat a lot less than usual even after going for a run.

*Make a point of screaming in pain if the candidate touches your cheeks without first asking for any pain. Also, make a point of blinking your eyes and rubbing them a lot during the conversation to draw the candidate's attention towards the fact that your eyes are dry and red.

Case 37 Task:	Achieved	Not Achieved
Introduces self, explains the goal of the encounter and acquires consent to proceed	███	
Demonstrates an infection-control compliant approach (bare below the elbows + clean hands before and after the examination)		
Makes a point of asking the patient for any painful / tender areas to be considerate towards these during examination		
Checks (personally or asks for) the patient's basic observations (temperature, BP, HR, RR, SaO2 on air). Comments on the pyrexia		
Inspection of the face and neck: Comments on the bilateral parotid swellings (looks between the sternocleidomastoid muscle and the mandible), and the lack of obvious swelling in the submandibular (between the angle of the mandible and the mylohyoid muscle) and sublingual regions (floor of the mouth/antero-inferior aspect of the chin) Looks for obvious skin abnormalities, scars or skin defects overlying the tract of the salivary ducts Inspects the oral cavity (with an appropriate light source), and uses tongue depressors to ensure a thorough inspection to include the openings of the six salivary ducts (parotid duct – opposite the upper 2nd molar teeth) Comments on the xerostomia, presence of food debris, ulcers on the tip of the tongue, the dental caries, and pus at the opening of the left parotid duct. Also mention the presence/absence of ductal stones) Comments on the kerato-conjuctivitis sicca and the relatively dry skin (patient not sweating)		
Palpation: Palpates the glands whilst standing behind the patient (elicits left sided tenderness) Examines the parotid swellings systematically looking for consistency (homo/heterogeneous), texture (firm/soft), fluctuancy, etc		

Assess for adherence to underlying structure by externally palpating the glands whilst the patient has their mouth opened, and then with the teeth clenched Externally milk the glands, assessing the fluid expressed from each duct. Comment on the pus from the left parotid duct, and the dryness of the other ducts Wearing gloves, palpate the glands bimanually (thumb inside the mouth, fingers outside), assessing the consistency of the glands, palpating for stones, and expression of pus/saliva (warn the patient before doing this)		
Assesses facial symmetry and muscle weakness (CN VII palsy)		
Carries out a comprehensive palpation of all neck regions (all 5 levels of the neck, thyroid gland, sub-clavicular, supra-clavicular, peri-auricular, TMJ's, occipital, and parotids), and systematically describes palpable masses (location, size, texture, mobility, tenderness, mobility)		
Suggests performing Schirmer's test to assess tear production		
Demonstrates good rapport and empathy with the patient throughout the encounter		
Relays a concise summary of findings to the examiner		
Expresses a wish to perform a full ENT examination		
Suggests investigations in a logical manner (1 mark for all 3 points): Lists required blood tests (blood film, FBC, LFT's, U&Es, LDH, infections serology, inflammatory markers, auto-antibodies – antinuclear antibodies, rheumatoid factor, SSA/Ro, SSb/La) FNAC USS / MRI / CT		
Examiner's Global Mark	/5	
Actor / Helper's Global Mark	/5	
Total Station Mark	/30	

Learning points:

- Salivary glands pathologies are relatively common, and most diagnoses can be made following a comprehensive history and examination of the glands and the fluid released from their ducts. The most sensitive aspect of the examination is direct palpation of the gland itself and assessing the nature of the fluid 'milked' via the duct

- Note that it is important to assess for facial nerve function as it is closely associated with the parotid gland Oral pathologies should be thoroughly assessed to exclude malignancies. It is also key to assess for lingual nerve function (tongue sensation and the sense of taste) as this lies in close proximity to the submandibular and sublingual glands.

- The diagnosis here is Sjögren's syndrome, with a complicating left sided (possible bacterial) parotitis. Other differentials include Sialolithiasis, infective/inflammatory causes (EBV/Mumps or other viral parotitis, Sarcoidosis), idiopathic (obesity, diabetes) and neoplastic (carcinomas, lymphoma, adenomas). Common neoplasms include pleomorphic adenomas, papillary cystadenoma (Warthin's tumor of the parotid), adenoid cystic carcinoma, squamous cell carcinoma, acinic cell tumors, etc.
  If a neoplastic process is suspected, a comprehensive oral, head & neck and general examination is crucial in order to evaluate the patient's lesion, and any spread in case of a suspected cancer. Please note that a comprehensive examination of the neck should include palpation of the lymph nodes in all '5 levels of the neck'; lymph nodes to in the submandibular, sub-clavicular, supra-clavicular, peri-auricular and occipital regions, the temporo-mandibular joints (TMJs) and thyroid gland.

Case 38

Candidate's instructions:

You are the Foundation doctor covering the medical wards on a night shift. The nurse on MAU has asked you to see Mr. J Peacock, an 85 year old gentleman who was admitted earlier in the day with a urinary tract infection. He is currently on 1.2g IV Co-Amoxiclav, TDS. The nurse's concern is to do with the funny sounds he's making with his breathing. Please **assess** this patient's airway.

You have 8 minutes for this station, but will get a warning bell 2 minutes prior to the end. Please use this remaining time to collect your thoughts and discuss any other important points you will like to cover.

Examiner's instructions:

The candidate has to rapidly assess a deteriorating patient from an airway point of view. You are assessing the candidate on their systematic approach in dealing with the patient, and the safety of the patient assessment.

Do not give the candidate any information unless specifically requested by the candidate. Guide the station in a direction where an anaesthetist is required, with the patient eventually being intubated.

The candidate has 8 minutes for this station, but please give them a warning with 2 minutes to go.

Patient Info:

85M, with a history of COPD. Penicillin allergic. Developed symptoms 15 minutes after the evening drug round.

Initial assessment:
A: Dyspnoea with stridor
B: Peripherally cyanotic (finger nails, toe-nails)
      Tachypnoea (Resp rate 34)
      Moderate bilateral air entry on auscultation
      Use of accessory respiratory muscles noted, with a marked effort of breathing
C: a flushed sweaty face
      distended neck veins + mild swelling on the anterior aspect of the neck
D: GCS E4 V3 M5
Further assessment:
A: Reduced stridor
B: Cyanosis involving the lips
      Resp rate 8
      Minimal air entry bilaterally
      reduced use of the accessory muscles, reduced chest movement
C: Nil change in neck swelling
D: GCS E2 V1 M4

Case 38 Task:	Achieved	Not Achieved
Introduces self		
Checks patient identity		
Washes / Gels hands/ Apron/ gloves		
Speaks to the patient, asking them a question. Ascertains lack of coherent response. Speaks to the nurse instead, taking a quick history to include the duration of symptoms, events around the onset of events, PMHx, DHx and allergies		
Inspects the face, mouth, nose. Opens the mouth, and looks in each nostril		
Listens to the breathing pattern		
Feels for breathing with the side of the face		
Combines the look, listen, feel technique. Correctly recognizes that the patient is peripherally cyanotic, that there is a small anterior neck swelling, and that the patient has stridor		
On auscultation, identifies the equal but reduced bilateral air entry		
Asks specifically for the respiratory rate, heart rate, oxygen saturations		
Applies high flow oxygen		
When asked about the clinical impression at this point, correctly suggests an upper airway obstruction causing the stridor		
Correctly suggests an anaphylactic reaction, and suggests that the patient will be managed as per ALS anaphylaxis protocols		
When the patient deteriorates further, identifies the need for a crash call immediately		
Suggests the need for anesthetist for airway management		
Remains calm under pressure and demonstrates good clinical judgment at all times		
Relays a concise summary to the examiner		
Maintains professionalism at all times		
Shows an understanding of simple airway maneuvers such as the chin lift, jaw thrust, head tilt		

Discusses airway adjuncts such as an oropharyngeal (Guedel) airway and Nasopharyngeal airways; and the contraindication – skull base defect – for the latter		
Discusses the escalation of airway management re laryngeal masks, endotracheal tubes and surgical airways (tracheostomy, crico-thyroidectomy etc)		
Examiner's Global Mark	/5	
Actor / Helper's Global Mark	/5	
Total Station Mark	/30	

Key Learning points:

- Stridor is an acute airway emergency and should be treated as such. The patient must be assessed in the same systematic way of any other acutely unwell patient following the principles of an Airway, Breathing, Circulation protocol.

- Once stridor is noted, high flow oxygen via a non-rebreathe mask should be applied immediately. An airway specialist (anaesthetist +/- ENT specialist on-call) should be contacted immediately

- Ascertaining the cause of stridor should be the next immediate objective. This will help guide treatment, and in situations where the patient cannot maintain their own airway, adjuncts can be used initially, with the knowledge that this may well progress to a definitive airway; endotracheal or surgically (cricothyroidectomy/tracheostomy)

Case 39

Candidate's instruction:

You the medical foundation doctor on-call, and have been called to urgently assess this patient's tracheostomy. The patient is a 55 year-old man with a tracheostomy tube in-situ, inserted as part of a post endotracheal tube weaning process (long term intubated ITU patient)

Talk the assessor through the assessment and management steps you would take. Further clinical information may be given if requested.

You have 8 minutes for this station, but will get a warning bell 2 minutes prior to the end. Please use this remaining time to collect your thoughts and discuss any other important points you will like to cover.

Examiner's instruction:

Set up a mannikin with a tracheostomy tube in situ with tapes or Velcro ties to secure its position. The patient has a tracheostomy due to bilateral vocal cord palsy and recurrent aspiration pneumonia. The tracheostomy tube is size 7, double lumen, the cuff is inflated and the tube is non-fenestrated. The inner tube is blocked by a simulated mucous plug. A suction catheter, spare inner tube and spare tracheostomy tube must be available. Gloves and a visor should also be at the bedside. A flexible endoscope is not available during the scenario.

If requested, the observations at the start of the scenario are:

Pulse 108bpm, BP 146/76, RR 28, SpO2 87%. (Baseline SpO2 97%) **Each minute that passes without adequate intervention, the SpO2 falls by 2%. Relay the dropping SpO2 to the candidate

The cause of the problem is blockage of the inner tube by a mucous plug. A suction catheter will not pass through the trache tube. Deflating the cuff, applying O2 to the face and tracheostomy tube will stabilize the SpO2 and removing/replacing the inner tube will allow the SpO2 to rise and respiratory rate to normalize.

Replacing the tracheostomy tube completely or suggesting oral endotracheal intubation would stabilize the patient but global marks should be reduced to reflect the missed opportunity for simple 'first line' intervention.

The candidate has 8 minutes for this station, but please give them a warning with 2 minutes to go.

Case 39 Task:	Achieved	Not Achieved
Introduces self & clarifies who they are speaking to		
Uses PPE appropriately (Gloves, apron, visor etc)		
Identify airway compromise as an emergency situation		
Refers to ALS/ATLS guidelines		
Call for senior help (senior nurse, senior doctor, anesthetist or crash team all acceptable)		
Asks for SpO2 level or "observations"		
Applies high flow oxygen (15L/min) via trache mask to neck		
Deflates cuff of tracheostomy tube		
Applies high flow oxygen via non re-breathe face mask		
Assesses the position of the tube. i.e: tapes secure (2 fingers), tube sitting at normal angle		
Attempts suction of the tracheostomy tube		
Identifies that the suction catheter does not pass beyond the tip of the tracheostomy tube		
Removes inner tube		
Identifies blockage of the inner tube		
Replaces inner tube with a clean spare		
Auscultates chest to ensure adequate air entry		
Considers other causes of dyspnoea (eg: infection, thromboembolus, myocardial infarction)		
Recommends measures to prevent further mucous plugging (eg: humidified O2, saline nebulisers or a Heat and Moisture Exchange (HME) device)		
Projects an air of confidence throughout the station		
Demonstrates and ensures patient safety at all times (i.e calls for help asap, applies oxygen, attempts suction)		
Examiner's Global Mark	/5	
Actor / Helper's Global Mark	/5	
Total Station Mark	/30	

Key Learning points:

- An acutely dyspnoeic patient with a tracheostomy tube must be assessed in the same systematic way of any other patient following the principles of an Airway, Breathing, Circulation protocol. Remember that a patient with a tracheostomy has 2 airways to consider as they may well have a partially patent and useful upper airway. Therefore, apply oxygen to both. This is in contrast with a patient who has undergone a laryngectomy who is completely dependent on 'neck breathing'.

- There are many types of tracheostomy tube made from various materials and each has individual advantages. The important features of any tracheostomy tube to identify are its size, how it is positioned and secured, whether it has a cuff (inflated or not), fenestrations and is it a single or double lumen tube?

- Deflating the cuff will allow the patient to breathe around a blocked tube and should be considered immediately unless there is active bleeding that may be aspirated. Removing the inner tube should always be considered and a clean spare should be at the side of every patient.
    - The tracheostomy stoma tract is usually well formed after 2 weeks and sometimes the best or only option is to remove the tracheotomy tube altogether and hold the stoma open with tracheal dilating forceps, which should be in an emergency bag carried by every tracheostomy patient.

Case 40 - Data interpretation

Candidate Instruction:

You are the FY1 on nights. The outgoing day FY1 asks you to check some bloods on a 35 year old lady, who has just been admitted onto the cardiology ward. Unfortunately, the FY1 doesn't know much about the patient as the registrar saw her. All she knows is that she came in with a fast heart rate and was haemodynamically unstable but has recovered before being transferred to the cardiology ward.

On arrival at the cardiology ward you are presented blood results. Describe any abnormalities and answer the **six questions** from the examiner.

You have 8 minutes for this station, but will get a warning bell 2 minutes prior to the end. Please use this remaining time to collect your thoughts and discuss any other important points you will like to cover.

Bloods

WBC	3.9	4.0-11.0	Ca	2.30	2.12-2.65
Hb	100	115-160	Phosphate	1.12	0.8-1.25
Neut	3.2	2.0-7.5			
MCV	84	76-96			

Na	139	135-145	LFTs	pending
K	4.0	3.5-5.3		
U	3.5	2.5-6.7		
Cr	82	70-150		

TSH	<0.01	0.5-5.7
T3	15	3.5-7.8
T4	29	9.0-25.0

Examiners instruction:

The FY1 on nights has been handed over to check blood results on a patient that was admitted earlier in the day. They know only that the patient had a fast heart rate and was haemodynamically stable on arrival but they have now recovered and been admitted to the cardiology ward.

They will describe any abnormalities in the bloods and answer your following questions:

1. Makes a diagnosis based on the thyroid function tests.

2. Why is the TSH low?

3. What cardiac rhythm do you suspect the patient was admitted with?

4. Give five symptoms of hyperthyroidism (1 mark for each).

5. Give five signs of hyperthyroidism (1 mark for each).

6. What is Grave's disease

7. What three symptoms are found in Graves Disease only compared to hyperthyroidism?

The candidate has 8 minutes for this station, but please give them a warning with 2 minutes to go.

Case 40 Task:	Achieved	Not Achieved
Introduces self & clarifies who they are speaking to		
Bloods		
Notes normocytic anaemia. Offers heavy periods as a possible explanation Notes low TSH and elevated T3 & T4 levels		
Questions (1-7)		
Hyperthyroidism		
Raised T3/T4 causes negative feedback of the Hypothalamus-Pituitary-Thyroid pathway		
Atrial Fibrillation		
Suggests five symptoms: Unintentional weight loss Increased appetite Heat intolerance Tremors Dysmenorrhoea		
Suggests 5 signs: Goitre Thyroid bruit Tachycardia/Atrial Fibrillation Fine tremor Warm peripheries/Palmar erythema		
Explains that it is an autoimmune condition, in which thyroid stimulating hormone (TSH) receptor antibody is secreted, leading to a molecular mimicry in which the thyroid gland is hyperstimulated, resulting in the overproduction of the thyroid hormone (T3/T4)		
Suggests all three points: Ophthalmopathy (exophthalmos, ophthalmoplegia, chemosis, croneal ulceration) Pretibial myxedema Thyroid acropachy		
Examiner's Global Mark	/10	
Total Station Mark	/30	

Learning Points:

- The handover in this scenario is poor and in real practice it is important to know the whole story and why the bloods have been done. This is essential for patient safety and will save you time when you come to review the patient. In the context of this scenario, the cardiac manifestations of thyroid diseases can present acutely. Such presentations could lead to life threatening complications (Acute cardiac failure, arrhythmias, embolic events, thyroid storm). Therefore, suspected systemic acute complications should be addressed promptly and systematically, and should warrant an urgent referral for a medical expert opinion.

- Other signs include of hyperthyroidism include:
    - Proximal myopathy
    - Hyper-reflexia
    - Hair thinning
    - Lid lag/ophthalmoplegia
    - Clubbing
    - Anxiety/restlesness etc

- Patients with known thyroid disease can have distorted thyroid function when they become acutely unwell, and interpreting their blood results can be fraught with difficulty in an acute setting.

Section 4

Ophthalmology

Case 41

Candidate's instructions:

You are a Foundation doctor in the emergency department. You have been asked to see Agnes, an 85 year old lady who has been brought into the department complaining of loss of vision. She has no referral letter and hasn't been to the hospital before. Take a history, present your findings, suggest potentially useful investigations and a differential diagnosis.

After 6 minutes the examiner will stop you and ask you to summarise back your findings, suggest your management plan and answer some direct questions.

Examiner's instructions:

This is a station where the candidate has to elicit a history from a patient with monocular vision loss.

After 6 minutes, please stop the candidate and ask:

"Please summarise your findings and discuss how you would like to investigate and manage this patient."

Actors instruction:

You are an 84 year old lady with a 2 hour history of complete loss of vision in the left eye.

This morning whilst having coffee with your daughter, you noticed a sudden loss of vision in the left eye. 'Like the light switch was turned off in the room, but just with one eye'. You can only see the difference between light and dark. It has stayed like this since it began about 2 hours ago so you have been brought into the emergency department straight away by your daughter.

There were no preceding flashes of light or floaters in the eye and your other eye is completely fine. There is no pain in the left eye and no double vision, but you have had a headache for the past few days. It starts from the left temple, and radiates to the jaw and scalp. It is a dull ache that isn't really helped by either paracetamol or ibuprofen, it's there all the time and it is made worse when you have something to eat. Yesterday you had a couple of similar episodes, however they only lasted 30 seconds or so, so you ignored it.

No past problems with your eyes with the exception of having both cataracts removed 10 years ago. "In my younger days I was a bit short sighted but since I've had my cataracts done, I only need to wear my glasses for reading". You've been feeling generally run down for the past 6 weeks with aches and pains over the shoulders and back of the neck. Combing your hair has been more of an effort and when you get the brush on your scalp it has been a bit sore. "If you'd asked me a couple of months ago how my general health was I'd have said I was fit as a fiddle, but over the past few months I've been really feeling my age, with aches and pains and feeling generally run down." You haven't seen your GP about this.

No regular medications. You are allergic to penicillin – years ago it caused a rash.

You live alone, don't drive and are independent with activities of daily living.

Your mother was blind in one eye in later life but you don't know the cause. All children and grandchildren have normal, healthy eyes.

Your primary concern is that your symptoms are due to a stroke. Your sister recently died following a stroke. "Will I get my sight back?"

Case 41 task:	Achieved	Not Achieved
Introduces self & clarifies who they are speaking to		
History of presenting complaint. Specifically: Monocular / binocular Onset of symptoms Redness of eye Pain/photophobia Current level of vision		
Associated ocular symptoms. Specifically: Double vision Preceding amaurosis		
Associated systemic symptoms: Fatigue Jaw claudication Scalp tenderness		
Headache history SOCRATES plus red flags 2 from (nausea, vomiting, postural variation, morning onset)		
Past ophthalmic history (including refraction – Short sighted)		
Past family/medical/drug history + allergy status		
Explores Ideas, concerns, and expectations		
Demonstrates good rapport and empathy with the patient		
Relays a concise summary to the examiner		
Suggests any 2 useful investigations from (1 mark only) ESR/CRP (inflammatory markers) Full blood count ECG		
Offers differential diagnosis (1 mark only) Giant cell arteritis / Temporal arteritis (arteritic ischaemic optic neuropathy Non arteritic anterior ischaemic optic neuropathy (i.e. embolic event)		
Examiner's Global Mark	/5	
Actor / Helper's Global Mark	/5	
Total Station Mark	/30	

Learning Points:

- It is important to ask about specific symptoms e.g. photophobia, trauma, swelling, contact lens use as negatives can rule help rule out differentials.

- Always ask about driving when taking an ophthalmology history. If you don't one day it will catch you out. Guidelines state that patients must have a visual acuity of 6/12 or better (with contact lenses or glasses if necessary) using both eyes together or in the only eye if monocular.

- Asking about patients' ideas, concerns and expectations is especially important in ophthalmology. Sight is arguably the most important sense in humans, and the loss of vision can be a very debilitating disability, both physically and mentally. It is therefore important to demonstrate empathy towards patients' concerns, whilst and exploring their concerns and expectations.

Case 42

Candidate Instruction:

A 45-year-old gentleman has presented to eye casualty with right sided eye pain and redness. You are the Ophthalmology Foundation doctor in eye casualty and have been asked to take a concise history from the patient, and present the case to the registrar.

After 6 minutes the examiner will stop you and ask you to summarise back your findings, suggest your management plan and answer some direct questions.

Examiner instructions:

This is a station where the candidate has to elicit a history from a patient with right sided eye pain.

Ask the candidate to summarize their findings and suggest investigations and if there is time a differential diagnosis.

After 6 minutes, please stop the candidate and ask:

"Please summarise your findings and discuss how you would like to investigate and manage this patient."

Actors Instruction:

You are a 45-year old gentleman who over the last two days has developed pain and redness in the right eye. The pain has gradually been getting worse and described as an ache. It is much worse when you look at lights and so you have been wearing dark glasses. The pain does not radiate and nothing helps except the dark glasses. The eye has been watering more than usual but there is no discharge. The vision is blurry on the right side but you can still read large print. You don't wear contact lenses or glasses.

You have a past medical history of ulcerative colitis and lower back pain. You have also found that you have been walking with a stoop, which has gotten worse over the past 5 years. You have no allergies and take ibuprofen PRN when the pain in your back gets unbearable.

There is no family history, you don't smoke and live at home with your wife.

Your wife is going on holiday with friends for the first time in years and you will be looking after your two children all week. You are particularly worried if the eye is contagious, as you don't want to spread it to your children. If it is contagious your wife says she will cancel her trip and stay at home.

Case 42 Task:	Achieved	Not Achieved
Introduces self & clarifies who they are speaking to		
Asks open questions		
Takes a structured pain history using e.g SOCRATES		
Checks if symptoms are uni/bilateral		
Specifically asks about: Vision (blurred, dimmed, distorted, missing) Photophobia Foreign body History of trauma Grittiness/Itching Discharge Redness Glasses/ Contact Lenses Driving		
Asks about past Ophthalmic History		
Asks about past medical/surgical history/drug history and allergy status		
Asks about Family/Social History		
Explores Ideas, concerns, and expectations		
Demonstrates good rapport and empathy with the patient throughout		
Makes the connection between the back pain & stoop (ankylosing spondilitis), Ulcerative colitis and anterior uveitis as the main differential diagnosis		
Relays a concise summary to the examiner		
Examiner's Global Mark	/5	
Actor / Helper's Global Mark	/5	
Total Station Mark	/30	

Learning Points:

- This station highlights the importance of asking open questions and listening to all the 'vague' symptoms to fit everything together to make a diagnosis. It is very tempting to rush straight into SOCRATES when you hear pain.

- Remember that asking about past medical history, family history, social and drug history is important but is not just for completeness; It can give important clues to the diagnosis. In this case, exploring the past medical history will give certain clues as to a possible history of ankylosing spondylitis, which when combined with the Ulcerative colitis can suggest anterior uveitis as the main differential here.

- Always ask about driving when taking an ophthalmology history. If you don't one day it will catch you out. Guidelines state that patients must have a visual acuity of 6/12 or better (with contact lenses or glasses if necessary) using both eyes together or in the only eye if monocular.

Case 43

Candidate Instruction:

A 60-year-old lady has presented to eye casualty with redness in her eye. You are the Ophthalmology Foundation doctor in eye casualty and have been asked to take a history and then present the case to the registrar. You will also be expected to suggest possible differentials and a brief management plan.

After 6 minutes the examiner will stop you and ask you to summarise back your findings, suggest your management plan and answer some direct questions.

Examiner instructions:

A 60-year-old lady has presented to eye casualty with redness in her eye.
The candidate has been asked to take an initial history and present back the findings to the registrar.

After 6 minutes, please stop the candidate and ask:

"Please summarise your findings and discuss how you would like to investigate and manage this patient."

Actors Instruction:

You are a 60-year-old lady who over the last three hours has gradually developed redness and severe pain in your right eye. You glanced at the eye in the mirror earlier and noticed that it was red in the white area and that the pupil looked an odd shape. The pain feels like it is in the eye, is stabbing in nature, the worst you have ever had, makes you extremely sick and you feel you may vomit. You are not sensitive to light, there is no radiation and nothing has made it worse or better. You have noticed haloes around lights and the vision in the eye is blurry, much worse than normal even with your glasses on (you are long-sighted). The left eye is unaffected.

You are normally fit and well but have been taking antihistamines over the last few days for hay-fever. You have never smoked, do not drink alcohol and have no allergies.

You are extremely worried about the blurry vision, as you have been asked to drive your granddaughter to church for her wedding at the weekend.
*Expect a show of empathy, at this stage, and do not volunteer this information unless specifically asked about your ideas, concerns and expectations.

Case 43 Task:	Achieved	Not Achieved
Introduces self & clarifies who they are speaking to		
Checks if redness is : Unilateral Did symptoms start in one eye, before affecting the other?		
Takes a history re the vision Visual loss sudden or gradual Transient/ ongoing Blurred, dimmed, distorted, missing Haloes around lights Photophobia		
Specifically asks about: Pain (SOCRATES) Discharge from the eye (s) Grittiness/itching/swelling Foreign body/trauma Glasses/Contact Lens use Implications on driving		
Asks about past ophthalmic history		
Asks about drug history and allergies		
Asks about past medical/surgical/family/social history and allergies		
Explores Ideas, concerns, and expectations (This point can be gained if the candidate explores the patient's concerns re driving her granddaughter to the wedding)		
Demonstrates good rapport and empathy with the patient throughout		
Relays a concise summary to the examiner		
Examiner's Global Mark	/5	
Actor / Helper's Global Mark	/5	
Total Station Mark	/30	

Learning Points:

- A red eye can range from a simple conjunctivitis to sight threatening angle closure glaucoma or endophthalmitis. It is therefore important to take a detailed history. Visual acuity is the most important factor.

- It is important to ask about specific symptoms e.g. photophobia, trauma, swelling, contact lens use as negatives can rule help rule out differentials.

- Always ask about driving when taking an ophthalmology history. If you don't one day it will catch you out. Guidelines state that patients must have a visual acuity of 6/12 or better (with contact lenses or glasses if necessary) using both eyes together or in the only eye if monocular.

Case 44

Candidate Instruction:

A 24-year old lady has presented with right sided blurry vision. You are the Ophthalmology Foundation doctor in eye casualty and have been asked to take a focused **history and perform ishihara charts, pupillary response and fundoscopy.** Present your findings to the registrar following the examination.

After 6 minutes the examiner will stop you and ask you to summarise back your findings, suggest your management plan and answer some direct questions.

Examiner instructions:

A 24-year old lady has presented with right sided blurry vision. The candidate has been asked to take a focused history and examination.

After 6 minutes, please stop the candidate and ask:

"Please summarise your findings and discuss how you would like to investigate and manage this patient."

Examination findings:

Right		Left
Right		**Left**
6/36	Visual Acuity (unaided)	6/6
6/36	Visual Acuity (pinhole)	6/6
3/17	Colour Vision	17/17
Equal	Pupil inspection	Equal
Reacts slowly	Pupillary reaction	Normal reaction
Normal	Red reflex	Normal
Normal	Retina	Normal
Pale, swollen	Optic disc	Normal

Normal accommodation bilaterally

Right relative afferent pupillary defect (RAPD) - on shining light into right eye the pupil dilates. Light shone into the left eye causes pupillary constriction.

Actors Instruction:

You are a 24-year old lady who over the last couple of days has noticed gradual blurring of the right vision. You can still read large signs but struggle with reading smaller print.

The eye has also become slightly painful on eye movements there is no discharge or trauma.

You have never had anything like this in the past. You are otherwise fit, take no regular medications, have no allergies, no family history and do not smoke or drink.

Case 44 Task:	Achieved	Not Achieved
Introduces self & clarifies who they are speaking to		
History:		
Checks if symptoms are uni/bilateral		
Asks the following about vision: Blurred/dimmed/distorted Diplopia Onset of visual loss (sudden/insidious) Timing of visual loss (transient/ongoing)		
Specifically asks about: Photophobia Pain - SOCRATES		
Examination:		
Using snellen chart assesses visual acuity With Pinhole Without Pinhole		
Tests colour vision with Ishihara plates Tests each eye separately		
Inspects pupils		
Tests accomodation		
Darkens room and asks patient to fix on distant object Tests direct and consensual pupillary reactions Performs swinging light test		
Indicates ideally patient's eyes should be dilated Tests red reflex using fundoscope Examines retina using fundoscope		
Demonstrates good rapport with the patient throughout		
Guides the patient through the examination		
Relays a concise summary to the examiner		
Examiner's Global Mark	/5	
Actor / Helper's Global Mark	/5	
Total Station Mark	/30	

Learning Points:

- Differential Diagnoses
    - Inflammatory – **Optic Neuritis**, autoimmune disease, sarcoid
    - Ischemic – arteritic or non-arteritic ischaemic optic neuropathy
    - Nutritional – B12, folate, alcohol
    - Compressive – optic nerve, orbital or intracranial tumours
    - Systemic – severe hypertension, raised intracranial pressure

- If a patient wears glasses, ensure that they wear them when checking visual acuity and colour vision. Don't forget to test each eye individually.
  If a patient cannot see any letters on a snellen chart check the vision in the following order: counting fingers, hand movements, perception of light. Learn and practice how to use a fundoscope prior to the exam. There is nothing worse than stressing and wasting time in the exam trying to turn it on!

- The swinging light test is to check for a relative afferent pupillary defect. Shine the light in one eye for 3 seconds, then move the other for the same interval. Repeat as needed but do not spend longer on one eye than the other as this can bleach the retina and cause an artificial RAPD. If the right optic nerve is damaged, shining the light in the right eye will produce a normal efferent response in the left and right pupil. Moving to the right eye then causes a paradoxical dilation of both pupils as the stimulus is effectively diminished. A patient may tell you the light seems dimmer.

Case 45

Candidate's instruction:

You are the Foundation doctor on general medicine night duty. You are paged to your ward to see Bettie a 60-year old lady who complains of double vision of sudden onset. The patient was admitted with urosepsis which is resolving. She was switched to oral antibiotics yesterday and is waiting to go home tomorrow morning. Examine the relevant cranial nerves in the allotted time. You are not required to carry out any history taking.

After 6 minutes the examiner will stop you and ask you to summarise back your findings, suggest your management plan and answer some direct questions.

Examiner's instructions:

When the patient is being examined give the appropriate clinical findings if the candidate performs the correct examination technique or describes what they would like to do to elicit a clinical sign.
After 6 minutes, please stop the candidate and ask:

"Please summarise your findings and discuss how you would like to investigate and manage this patient."

Examination findings:

Observations
Comfortable at rest on room air
Resp 15, SpO2 98% on room air
Pulse 90, BP 128/79 Capillary refill time 3 seconds, Warm peripheries
36.5°C
GCS 15

Inspection
Normal head position
No proptosis
Left ptosis
When candidate lifts the upper lid the following signs are able to be seen:
Anisocoria (left pupil larger than right)
Left eye depressed and abducted when right eye looking straight ahead (patient complains of double vision when looking straight ahead)

Ocular Motility

Right eye –   Normal range of motion
Left eye   –   Normal abduction
             Restricted adduction.
             Restricted elevation
             Limitation of depression

Case 45 task:	Achieved	Not Achieved
Introduces self & clarifies who they are speaking to		
Washes / Gels hands		
Checks for any pain or discomfort before commencing examination		
Inspects patient and comments on head position		
Looks for proptosis		
Inspects patient in primary position Notes ptosis Notes anisocoria Notes deviated position of left eye when right eye in primary position		
Tests Abduction (Cranial nerve VI)		
Tests Cranial nerve IV (depression in abduction)		
Tests Cranial nerve III: Elevation Depression Adduction Adduction and depression in adduction		
Demonstrates good rapport and empathy with the patient		
Relays a concise summary to the examiner		
Offers differential diagnosis: 3rd nerve palsy, Cerebrovascular accident etc.		
Management plan:		
Needs urgent CT head		
Neurological observations		
Examiner's Global Mark	/5	
Actor / Helper's Global Mark	/5	
Total Station Mark	/30	

Learning points:

- If a patient wears glasses ensure that they wear them when checking visual acuity. Don't forget to test each eye individually.

- A good tip when testing for eye movements is to hold on to the patient's chin with your non-dominant hand (whilst drawing an exaggerated 'H' with dominant hand), to prevent hem from moving their head. Patient's can find a hand placed on their head not only uncomfortable, but also intimidating. Always explain to patients what you intend to do and why before laying hands on them.

- Assessing the patient's head position can give clues as to a cranial nerve lesion as the head is held in acertain way to overcome the effect of gravity on the function of specific extra-ocular muscles; for example, patients often tilt their head forward (chin tucked in) and to the opposite side to a IVth nerve palsy.

Case 46 - Data interpretation

Candidates instruction:

You are the Foundation doctor in general surgery. You are paged to your ward to see Mr. Smith a 58 year old man who complains of a painful left eye. The patient was admitted with biliary colic which is resolving.

Overnight, the patient has complained of an increasing dull ache pain in the left eye, which has been intensifying all day. There hasn't been any purulent discharge, but the patient has noticed increased tearing of his left eye.
He has had poor vision in that eye for many years, but in the past 24 hours has noted a decrease in vision.

Inspect the patient's medications and look at the picture overleaf of Mr. Smith's left eye.

After 6 minutes the examiner will stop you and ask you to summarise back your findings, suggest your management plan and answer some direct questions.

Patients medications
G. Maxidex- BD,
Acyclovir – BD,
Hypromellose - QDS

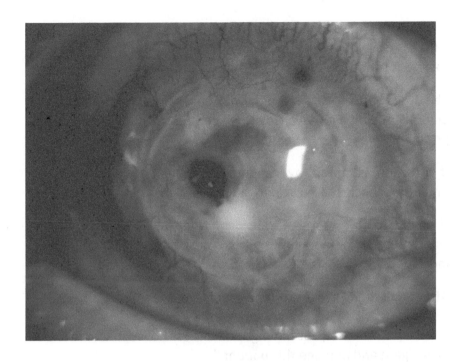

Examiner's instructions:

The picture shows a patient who has had a corneal transplant and who has developed an infection in the graft. This infection has led to a perforation in the centre of the cornea and prolapse of the iris.

The drug chart shows a steroid eye drop, artificial tears an oral and an oral antiviral agent Acyclovir (which is to maintain their corneal graft.

If infection is noted by candidate, ask about likely causative organisms (bacterial, viral, parasitic).

If candidate notes corneal transplant, and there is time remaining ask if they know about different types of transplant and their indications.

After 6 minutes, please stop the candidate and ask:

"Please summarise your findings and discuss how you would like to investigate and manage this patient."

If candidate is doing well and has time, ask about what the ophthalmic team are likely to do with the patient.

Case 46 Task:	Achieved	Not Achieved
Introduces self & clarifies who they are speaking to		
Notes conjunctival injection		
Notes corneal transplant		
Notes vascularization of cornea		
Notes corneal infiltrate		
Notes perforation of cornea		
Notes prolapse of iris		
Notes flat anterior chamber		
Notes sutures (on close inspection of the picture)		
Comments on Acyclovir on drug chart		
Infers that corneal graft was probably due to herpetic keratitis		
Relays a concise summary of clinical findings to the examiner		
Offers diagnosis: Perforation corneal graft ? due to infection(microbial keratitis)		
Management plan: Immediate discussion with on-call ophthalmologist Analgesia Cover the eye with a shield (or don't touch the eye)		
Knowledge of ophthalmic management: Antibiotics - Topical Bandage contact lens New corneal graft		
Examiner's Global Mark	/10	
Total Station Mark	/30	

Learning points:

- The picture shows an obvious perforation of the corneal graft. This is, clearly an ophthalmic emergency and prompt management may salvage sight, or prevent loss of the eye altogether.

- If you encounter a situation like this, ask for help from a senior colleague. Do not touch the eye, and try to encourage the patient to leave their eye alone. If it is possible, try to find an eye shield (they are available from eye theatres).

- If the perforation is amenable to temporizing measures, a corneal gluing procedure may be performed in theatres or the outpatients' clinic. In this case, treatment of the causative microbial keratitis was necessary before definitive treatment. This involved siting of a bandage contact lens and high frequency topical antibiotics. Definitive management options include re-do corneal transplant, a patch graft or covering the cornea with a flap of conjunctiva.

Section 5
Advanced communication skills

Case 47
Candidates instructions:

You are a Foundation doctor on an Ophthalmology ward, and you've been asked by your consultant, to speak to a 65-year old patient who had just been transferred to the eye day unit from recovery after a routine cataract surgery that morning.

You are in a difficult situation as you were involved in the case and it was only after the operation that you realize you have operated on the wrong eye. The patient was admitted for surgery on the left eye, but due to an unexplainable and catastrophic error, the patient's 'right' eye was operated on.

Your consultant is back in theatres operating on a big case that will take hours to complete. He has asked you to talk to the patient, explain what happened during the operation, and deal with any immediate queries.

The consultant will see the patient after his case, and deal with any unanswered questions.

As the patient has a tremor the operation was undertaken under general anaesthetic rather than the usual local. You go and see him once the anaesthetic has worn off.

Your task during this encounter is to deliver the difficult news to the patient and respond to the patient's concerns. The station should take 8 minutes in total, with a warning bell 2 minutes prior to the end, and the last 1 minute to summarise and conclude the conversation appropriately.
Examiner's Instructions:

This is a complex case, however the crux of the case is the appropriate breaking of bad news. The candidate has to do this in a sensitive way, but be mindful of the time limitation of the station and their own lack of detailed specialist knowledge.

The station should take 8 minutes in total, with a warning bell 2 minutes prior to the end, and the last 1 minute to summarise and conclude the conversation appropriately.

Actors instructions:

You are a 65 year-old gentleman who has just returned to the eye day unit after having cataract surgery. The surgery was undertaken under general anaesthetic as you have a tremor. The operation was on the right eye but you have an eye shield over the left eye, which has already started you thinking that something is amiss.

The junior doctor you met earlier has come to talk to you. The doctor will explain that the left eye was operated on by mistake.

During the consultation, in no particular order, you should mention.

You are shocked. How could this happen? Surely there are safeguards to prevent this from happening.

You are livid as the left eye vision was very good before and now it has been operated on. Will the vision in the left eye be as good as it was before?

When will the consultant come and talk to you? Demand to speak to him now.

If they mention anything about operating on the right eye say that there is no chance of you visiting the hospital again.

You want to speak to someone to make a formal complaint.

You are a self-employed artist and are worried that now the good eye has been operated on you won't be able to work. You had been struggling to paint for the last three months and was looking forward to having good vision again.

You demand to know whose individual fault it is.

Ask how the right eye could be operated on when there was no cataract. What was done in the operation?

You want to see the hospital notes. If the doctor will not allow it, ask him what is stopping him from changing them after this meeting.

You want reassurance that despite the wrong eye being operated on that the operation went well.

Case 47 Task:	Achieved	Not Achieved
Introduces self & clarifies who they are speaking to		
Checks if they will prefer anyone else in the room with them		
Clarifies how much the patient knows already		
Gives a warning shot		
Explains in simple terms that the wrong eye was operated on		
Apologies to the patient		
Allows patient to vent their frustrations and anger		
Gives patient appropriate time to ask questions		
Does not blame any individual		
Uses appropriate vocabulary during explanation		
Stays calm through the consultation		
Defuses situation with patient demanding to see consultant		
States that a critical incident form will be filled and a full investigation will occur		
Offers the services of PALS for an official complaint and support		
Is honest with the patient and doesn't offer anything that can't be done		
Explain that the patient can see the hospital notes but this has to be done through an official route		
Summarises what has been discussed and action to be taken		
Knows limits when pressed by the patient		
Checks ideas & concerns and expectations		
Demonstrates good rapport and empathy with the patient		
Examiner's Global Mark	/5	
Actor / Helper's Global Mark	/5	
Total Station Mark	/30	

Learning points:

- Admitting to a patient that a mistake has been made is terrifying. The most important thing is to be completely honest and we all should now adhere to the 'Duty of Candour' that the GMC recommends. The guidance says that doctors, nurses and midwives should:

    - - speak to a patient, or those close to them, as soon as possible after they realise something has gone wrong with their care
    - - apologise to the patient, explaining what happened, what can be done if they have suffered harm and what will be done to prevent someone else being harmed in the future
    - - report errors at an early stage so that lessons can be learned quickly, and patients are protected from harm in the future.

- The first meeting is crucial in establishing rapport. If a mistake has been made then it is likely this will not be the last time you see the patient. In fact you should see them more that you would a normal patient to make sure that nothing else can go wrong. If you start the first consultation on the wrong foot then every time you see the patient it will be more difficult.

Remember that you aren't alone in handling a mistake. PALS (patient advice and liaison service) is an essential team and should be offered to all patients who may want to make a formal complaint.

Case 48
Candidate's instructions:

You are a foundation doctor and the 'first on-call' for ENT on a night shift. You were called to the emergency department (ED) to urgently assess a child with an airway obstruction in the paediatric resuscitation unit. You, the on-call paediatric anaesthetist and paediatrician have assessed the patient and made the diagnosis of an airway obstruction that is caused by supraglottitis or severe croup.

The patient is a 4 year old girl who is previously fit and healthy. She has recently had a cold that progressed tonight into severe respiratory distress, drooling and noisy breathing. The examination findings are: fever, drooling, biphasic stridor, lethargy with irritability, tracheal tugging and inter-costal recession, and SaO2 of 85% on air. Further examination is avoided in order to avoid laryngeal spasm and complete airway obstruction. The symptoms improve slightly with steroids and nebulised adrenaline, but worsen shortly afterwards. The patient has received maximum wide-spectrum antibiotics and steroids doses, is on humidified maximum oxygen, and is observed closely in a quiet environment.

A multidisciplinary discussion has taken place between your on-call seniors (who are on the way to the hospital), the on-call paediatrician and paediatric anaesthetist. A final joint decision is made to transfer the child imminently to theatre to secure her airway through an endo-tracheal intubation +/- emergency tracheostomy, then to carry out a diagnostic endoscopy of the upper airway under general anaesthesia. The patient's father is away abroad but her mother is present and is extremely devastated and concerned regarding what her girl is going through.

Your task during this encounter is to deliver the difficult news regarding the diagnosis and management plan to the patient's parent. You are not required to take formal consent as this will be carried out by your seniors on their arrival.

The station should take 8 minutes in total, with a warning bell 2 minutes prior to the end, and the last 1 minute to summarise and conclude the conversation appropriately.

Examiner's instructions:

This is a communication skills scenario about breaking bad news to a child's parent. The child is a 4 year old girl who has severe airway obstruction that is due to severe croup / epiglottitis, and is not responding to intensive medical therapy. A multidisciplinary decision had been made to manage the child via an urgent endo-tracheal intubation +/- emergency tracheostomy and a diagnostic airway endoscopy under GA afterwards. The candidate is tasked to break the news to the child's mother who is extremely upset and worried. The diagnosis is already established and therefore the candidate does not require carrying out further examinations or history taking, and should be reminded of this as required. Also, the candidate is not required to take formal consent from the parent regarding the procedure. Your role during this scenario is purely an observant role; no intervention should be required from yourself.

The candidate is expected to approach such a difficult scenario professionally, empathically, and systematically.

The candidate should;
- Ensure that the scenario takes place in an appropriate environment.
- Express their preference to be supported by a nurse during the encounter in real life.
- Assess the parent's knowledge of events and ask for permission to provide information.
- Use a jargon-free progressive method of explaining the problem and management plan.
- Ensure that the mother understands the picture and that she is given Time to process the information and ask questions.
- Not shy away from admitting he/she will need to seek advice from his/her seniors should the parent ask a question he/she can't answer.

Finally, a summary should be provided by the candidate, and a future plan for communication should be explained.

The station should take 8 minutes in total, with a warning bell 2 minutes prior to the end, and the last 1 minute to summarise and conclude the conversation appropriately.

Actors instructions:

You are a 30 year old mother of a previously fit and healthy 4 year old girl; you have no other children and your husband is currently abroad. Your child has had a cold that worsened tonight as she started drooling and developed a difficult noisy breathing. Despite her being given many medicines, oxygen and nebulisers in the emergency department she remains unwell.

She has been assessed by many doctors and you are extremely worried and distressed. Tonight, you have seen your child becoming very unwell, witnessed her being exposed to various interventions, and now you are worried her life is at risk. You are wondering if you could have done something to stop her becoming very unwell. You don't know either whether or not the doctors at the emergency department have done everything they can to make her get better. On top of it, you have no idea as to what is the problem that is causing your daughter to be this poorly.

The candidate is one of the ear, nose and throat (ENT) doctors and is going to explain to you the diagnosis and management plan. He/she will explain to you that the problem is almost definitely an infection of the upper airway that is causing the airway to swell up and therefore become blocked. You could have done nothing different to stop this infection from progressing; the doctor should explain that to you. You will be told that your girl had failed to respond to various medical (conservative) extensive treatments at the emergency department. Therefore, the candidate should tell you that, your daughter requires an urgent invasive procedure to secure her airway and preserves her life.

The procedure, you will be told is an intubation (breathing tube through the mouth), a possible tracheostomy (breathing tube through a surgical opening in the neck), and an endoscopy of her airway to identify the exact cause of her symptoms. The candidate will explain to you that there is a risk to life during the procedure but that risk is far greater (definite) if no intervention is to take place. After the procedure your child will be looked after in the intensive care unit until it is deemed safe to remove the breathing tube and transfer her to the paediatric ward.

The candidate is expected to make sure you are happy with the environment and should preferably offer you the presence of one of the nurses / relatives / friends during the encounter to support you.

He/she should ask you about what you know is going on so far, and then asks for your permission for him/her to explain what the picture is.

The doctor should explain the problem / management in lay terms and in a progressive understandable manner.

The candidate should ensure your understanding of what is being said and keep checking if you have any queries.

At the end of the discussion, the candidate should construct a summary of what has been discussed and agreed and provide you with information on where to direct any further queries.

The candidate should be professional and empathetic. He/she should make you feel you are listened to, understood and reassured. They should respond to your emotions and reactions professionally, considerately and confidently. You should feel engaged in the process, able to ask questions, and to be provided with satisfactory answers.

The candidate should not shy away from admitting he/she will need to seek advice from his/her seniors should you ask a question he/she can't answer.

Case 48 Task:	Achieved	Not Achieved
Introduces self and explains objectives (e.g. "I would like to talk to you about your daughter's condition")		
Ensures that the scenario takes place within a safe quiet environment without interruptions		
Ensures that a member of the nursing team is available for support. Also asks if the parent prefers the presence of a relative or friend too.		
Asks open-ended questions to develop a good picture of what the parent knows so far, so the news is tailored to address their knowledge		
Assesses if the parent is willing to receive the offered information and how would they like to receive it		
Prepares the recipient for bad news by starting with phrases such as "I'm very sorry to say..." or "Unfortunately, I have to say..."		
Explains the diagnosis honestly and in non-medical terms		
Explains the condition can be fatal if not treated appropriately and vigorously		
Uses silent pauses to allow the recipient to process information and ask questions		
Explains what treatments have been administered so far and that they have proved ineffective		
Explains (in no jargon) that the best plan of action to preserve life ("... we need to secure her airway") is to imminently perform a procedure where "... we put her to sleep and pass a breathing tube"		
Explains the need for a diagnostic endoscopy under GA as this is crucial for further management		
Explains the possibility of failure to intubate which necessitates an emergency surgical tracheostomy		
Explains the stay in paediatric intensive care unit (PICU) stay postoperatively		

Delicately explains that although the procedure entails risk to life, the risk is far greater if the procedure is not carried out imminently		
Keeps checking for and addressing any queries, while using a nice flow of information in lay terms		
Responds to the recipient's reactions (tearfulness, silence or anger) professionally and empathetically by ensuring he/she lets the parent feel that he/she recognises, understands and responds to her feelings		
Asks for permission then summarise plan of action and progress of events (transfer to theatre, senior obtaining consent, procedure, postoperative care)		
Checks for any final queries, provides ways to contact someone to answer future queries and how further updates will be provided		
Admits inability to answer all questions and refers to seniors in order to attain answers		
Examiner's Global Mark	/5	
Actor / Helper's Global Mark	/5	
Total Station Mark	/30	

Learning points:

- Breaking bad news is an essential communication skill of all medical practitioners. On most occasions a senior doctor will be the one to break serious news, however doctors of all grades should have a structured approach to how to discuss difficult topics with patients and families. The delivery is as much, if not more important than the content.

- You should be professional, empathetic, and systematic when approaching a patient or parent to break bad news to them. Honesty is the key and do not be afraid to say you don't know all the precise details but will of course endeavour to find out and get back to them.

- One of the systems you can use in breaking bad news scenarios is a 6-step method referred to as "SPIKES"
    - Setting Up (environment / escort / nurse)
    - Assessing Perception (what do they know so far)
    - Obtaining Invitation (to give information)
    - Giving Knowledge (no jargon)
    - Emotions and Empathy (recognise / respond to their feelings)
    - Strategy and Summary (Assess understanding + future plan)

Case 49

Candidate's instructions:

You are a Foundation doctor in ENT, and are sitting in with your consultant at the head & neck outpatient clinic. The next patient is a 55 year old life-long smoker man who was seen in clinics two weeks ago with a 3X3cm right sided level III neck mass and, a right sided tonsillar enlargement. The examination on his previous appointment was otherwise normal and he was therefore referred to have an ultrasound (USS) guided fine needle aspiration (FNAC) of the mass, an MRI scan of the neck and a CT scan with contrast of the chest. The FNAC yielded metastatic squamous cell carcinoma (SCC). The head & neck multidisciplinary meeting (MDT) discussed the results and recommended that the patient should be investigated fully in order to identify the primary site of the metastatic cervical SCC. The chosen plan of action by the MDT to identify the primary site includes a PET-CT (Positron emission tomography-computerised tomography scan) and an urgent pan-endoscopy +/- biopsies +/- tonsillectomy under GA.

The patient is not aware that he has cancer and that the primary site is still to be confirmed. Also the patient is not aware of what the next step in his cancer diagnosis / management is going to be. Just before calling the patient in, the consultant got called to the emergency theatres for an urgent tracheostomy; you are now the only ENT doctor in clinic.

The station should take 8 minutes in total, with a warning bell 2 minutes prior to the end, and the last 1 minute to summarise and conclude the conversation appropriately.

Examiner's instructions:

This is a communication skills scenario where the candidate is expected to deliver bad news to an adult male patient in ENT outpatients. The patient is a 55 year old man who has a right sided metastatic neck SCC with, so far, an unknown primary. The patient's case was discussed at the head and neck MDT meeting and the plan is for him to have a pan-endoscopy +/- tonsillectomy and a PET-CT. The counselling is usually carried out by the consultant but the trainee will execute this task as the consultant is called for an emergency.

The candidate is tasked to break the news regarding the diagnosis and management plan to the patient. The patient is very anxious and is expecting to receive definitive answers regarding his condition having had several investigations already. The candidate is expected to counsel the patient regarding the diagnosis of a neck cancer with an unknown primary, the required further diagnostics, and the possible complications of the planned procedures.

The essential information that should be communicated includes:

- A diagnosis of cancer is yielded from the neck lump
- No known primary site of the metastatic cancer is found yet; every effort should be made to identify the primary site in order to construct the best treatment strategy
- A further new scan (PET-CT) is required as it can aid the identification of primary sites if not successfully visualised clinically
- Also, an endoscopy of the upper aero-digestive tract under GA is required to examine closely all areas that could conceal the primary site
- During the procedure, if no obvious abnormality is found to take a biopsy from, a tonsillectomy will be performed to rule out a microscopic intra-tonsillar primary cancer

- The surgical complications include pain, bleeding, and dental trauma. The diagnostic benefits outweigh the risks of surgery
- The final treatment modalities include surgery, radiotherapy, chemotherapy or various combinations of all three. The best combination varies according to the findings of all investigations and will be decided by the MDT pending the results
- The relevant contact details (especially the Head and Neck Specialist Nurse) to answer all questions throughout the journey should be provided to the patient

The diagnosis has already been established and therefore the candidate does not require carrying out further examinations or history taking, and should be reminded of this as required. Also, the candidate is not required to take formal consent from the patient regarding the procedure. Your role during this scenario is purely an observant role; no intervention should be required from yourself.

Points should be awarded according to how the candidate performs against the following standards in communication skills:
- The candidate ensures that the scenario takes place in an appropriate environment
- He/she expresses his/her preference to be supported by the Head and Neck Specialist Nurse during the encounter in real life
- The candidate apologises for the absence of the consultant and explains the emergency circumstances
- He/she assesses the patient's knowledge of the diagnosis and asks for his permission to provide information
- He/she uses a jargon-free progressive method of explaining the problem and management plan
- The candidate ensures that the patient understands the picture and is given time to process the information and ask questions

- He/she summarises the discussed diagnosis and management plan and advises on how to contact the team and Head & Neck Specialist Nurse
- The candidate does not shy away from admitting he/she will need to seek advice from the consultant when he/she can't provide an answer
- The candidate is overall professional, empathetic, and systematic

The station should take 8 minutes in total, with a warning bell 2 minutes prior to the end, and the last 1 minute to summarise and conclude the conversation appropriately.

Actors instructions:

You are a 55 year man who smoked for many years. You have been investigated for a lump on the right side of your neck in the ENT outpatients' department. You have had a needle biopsy, an MRI and a CT scan to investigate your lump. You are very anxious that this lump might be cancerous and are expecting, having had multiple investigations, to be given a definitive diagnosis and treatment plan from the specialists. You are met by the ENT doctor who will talk to you in outpatients.

The doctor will explain to you that he or she is one of the ENT doctors and that his/her consultant had to go to theatre to perform a lifesaving surgery. The candidate will explain to you that the lump in your neck was found to be cancerous. You will be told that this lump represents a spread from a cancer in your head and neck, but the primary cancer site is yet to be found. You will be told that the investigations you have had could not identify the primary site and therefore further investigations are required. The doctor will tell you that you need a different kind of a scan for the whole of your body (PET-CT).

Also you will be told that you need a total endoscopy under endoscopy under GA +/- biopsies of any abnormal looking areas. During the procedure, if no abnormality is to be identified, the surgeon will remove your tonsils in order to rule out an occult (microscopic) focus of cancer in them. The candidate will explain to you that the risks of surgery will include pain, trauma to teeth and a possibility of post-operative bleeding. You will be reassured that the diagnostic benefits of the procedure outweigh its risks. Pending the results of the scan and procedure, further management plan of your cancer will be decided at the multidisciplinary (MDT) meeting for head and neck cancers.

During the scenario of communicating bad news, you should expect that:

- The candidate will make sure you are happy with the environment and will offer you the presence of one of the nurses / relatives / friends to support you.
- He/she will ask you about what you know so far, and then ask for your permission to explain what the picture is
- The doctor will explain the problem / management in lay terms and in a progressive understandable manner
- The candidate will ensure your understanding of what is being said and keep checking if you have any queries
- At the end of the discussion, he/she will construct a summary of what has been discussed and provide you with information on where to direct any further queries (the Head and Neck Specialist Nurse)
- The candidate is professional and empathetic throughout the encounter. He/she will make you feel that you are listened to, understood and reassured. He/she will respond to your emotions and reactions professionally, considerately and confidently. You should feel engaged in the process, able to ask questions, and to be provided with satisfactory answers
- The candidate will not shy away from admitting that he/she will need to seek advice from the consultant if he/she does not know the answer to your queries

Case 49 Task:	Achieved	Not Achieved
Introduces self and explains objectives (e.g. "I would like to talk to you about the diagnosis and management plan of your neck lump")		
Ensures that the scenario takes place (or ask for that in a simulated scenario) within a safe quiet environment without interruptions		
Ensures that (or expresses preference in a simulated scenario) the specialist nurse is available for support, and asks if the patient prefers the presence of a relative or a friend		
Asks open-ended questions (e.g. "What do you know is going on so far?") to develop a good picture of what the patient / relatives know so far, so the news is tailored to address their knowledge		
Assesses if the patient is willing to receive the offered information and how would he like to receive it		
Prepares the recipient for bad news by starting with phrases such as "I'm very sorry to say" or "Unfortunately, I have to say", or "I'm afraid I have bad news"		
Gives the diagnosis in non-medical frank terms: "The investigations have confirmed that the lump in your neck is cancerous"		
Explains that the cancer in the lump is a spread (metastatic) from another area (the primary site) in the head and neck that is yet to be found		
Uses silent pauses to allow the recipient to process the information and ask questions		
Explains that identifying the primary cancer site is crucial in order to decide the best treatment plan		
Explains (in no jargon) that the best plan of action should be to make every effort in order to identify the primary site via a further scan and a procedure under general anaesthesia (GA)		
Explains that the PET-CT scan is very useful in picking up a small primary site from which the cancer might have spread to the neck node		

Explains the intended procedure as an endoscopy under GA +/- biopsies +/- tonsillectomy. Also, explains that a tonsillectomy is important if no primary site is to be found on endoscopy		
Explains that the procedure is a day case procedure under GA and can be associated with the risks of pain, bleeding and dental trauma		
Explains that the results will be discussed at the MDT meeting in order to construct the best treatment plan		
Keeps checking for and addressing any queries, while using a nice flow of information in lay terms		
Responds to the recipient's reactions (tearfulness / silence / anger) professionally and empathetically by letting the patient feel that he/she recognises, understands and addresses his feelings		
Asks for permission then summarises plan of action and progress of events (PET-CT, procedure, postoperative care, MDT plan following results)		
Checks for any final queries and provides details on how to contact the Head and Neck Specialist Nurse		
Admits inability to answer all questions and refers to seniors in order to attain answers		
Examiner's Global Mark	/5	
Actor / Helper's Global Mark	/5	
Total Station Mark	/30	

Learning points:

- Breaking bad news is an essential communication skill of all medical practitioners. On most occasions a senior doctor will be the one to break serious news, however doctors of all grades should have a structured approach to how to discuss difficult topics with patients and families. The delivery is as much, if not more important than the content.

- You should be professional, empathetic, and systematic when approaching a patient or parent to break bad news to them. Honesty is the key and do not be afraid to say you don't know all the precise details but will of course endeavour to find out and get back to them.

- One of the systems you can use in breaking bad news scenarios is a 6-step method referred to as "SPIKES"
    - Setting Up (environment / escort / nurse)
    - Assessing Perception (what do they know so far)
    - Obtaining Invitation (to give information)
    - Giving Knowledge (no jargon)
    - Emotions and Empathy (recognise / respond to their feelings)
    - Strategy and Summary (Assess understanding + future plan)

Case 50

Candidates instruction:

You are a Foundation doctor in Ophthalmology. You are seeing the new referrals in the outpatient clinic and your next patient is Captain Smith. He is a 49 year old airline pilot who has been referred to your clinic by their optometrist with a suspicious looking naevus on their right retina.

Your clinical examination has shown the lesion is highly suspicious of a choroidal melanoma. This is a malignant lesion which requires urgent attention, you therefore plan to refer the patient to the local tertiary centre. You have discussed the case with your consultant who agrees with your diagnosis and management plan.

The patient has a visual field defect which means Captain Smith would not meet the legal criteria to fly.

Due to the size of the lesion it is likely that surgery and / or radiotherapy is required. This treatment will permanently affect the vision in Captain Smith's right eye. This will mean Captain Smith is unable to pilot an aircraft.

Your task during this encounter is to deliver the difficult news to the patient and respond to the patient's concerns. The station should take 8 minutes in total, with a warning bell 2 minutes prior to the end, and the last 1 minute to summarise and conclude the conversation appropriately.

Examiner's Instructions:

This is a complex case, however the crux of the case is the appropriate breaking of bad news. The candidate has to do this in a sensitive way, but be mindful of the time limitation of the station and their own lack of specialist knowledge.

The station should take 8 minutes in total, with a warning bell 2 minutes prior to the end, and the last 1 minute to summarise and conclude the conversation appropriately.

Actors instructions:

You have been ignoring symptoms of new floaters in the right eye for some months because you are afraid of a diagnosis of any impairment of visual function affecting your ability to fly.

You are extremely anxious about the likely diagnosis of cancer.

You are initially disbelieving and shocked by the news you have cancer.

"You must have it wrong - I want to see the consultant" and you become increasingly insistent. When informed that the case has discussed and the supervising consultant who agrees with the findings of the investigations and the plan.

"Will this affect my job?" keep pressing until you have a direct answer.

After explaining that your diagnosis and subsequent treatment will affect the vision in your eye such that you are no longer able to fly, you become emotional.

"But what else can a 49 year old pilot do? - I've been flying all my working life"

How am I going to support my family? You are married and have three children, two of which are in a very expensive private boarding school as you often spend long periods away with work. You have no siblings and both your parents have died in the past year.

If the candidate is struggling to explain the intricacies of the condition, press them until they admit they don't know all the answers and they will find out and get back to you.

Case 50 Task:	Achieved	Not Achieved
Introduces self & clarifies who they are speaking to		
Clarifies how much the patient knows already		
Explains the diagnosis to the patient		
Uses the word 'cancer'		
Tells the patient they do not meet the requirements to fly		
Appropriate vocabulary during explanation		
Checks understanding		
Defuses situation with patient demanding to see consultant		
Explains the management plan: Referral to specialist centre Mentions radiotherapy Mentions surgery Explains that treatment will probably affect the patient's vision		
Pauses and give patient time to respond and ask questions with appropriate use of silence		
Assesses social situation and support		
Checks ideas & concerns and expectations		
Demonstrates good rapport and empathy with the patient		
Knows limits when pressed by the patient		
Appropriate closure of interview		
Offers written advice / copy of your letter		
Offers to contact other support services e.g. Macmillan or specialist nurses		
Examiner's Global Mark	/5	
Actor / Helper's Global Mark	/5	
Total Station Mark	/30	

Learning points:

- This scenario is designed to assess how you approach breaking bad news to a patient with the added complexity of dealing with the impact of a serious diagnosis of the patient's lifestyle. People are understandably defensive over their ability to drive or perform specialist occupations such as flying as is demonstrated in this case. Therefore, dealing with this situation sensitively is vital.

- Introduce yourself, check you know everyone in the room and how they are related to the patient and also make sure you introduce anyone else in the room, such as nursing staff or medical students. Prepare the environment if possible: ensure you are not interrupted, use a quiet room and if possible, get a colleague to hold your bleep. Having knowledge of the relevant facts surrounding the care of the patient, such as test results etc. Also, make sure you have a plan for what you would like to do with the patient.

- Know your limits and do not be afraid of admitting you don't know something. It is much better to admit your lack of knowledge, and tell the patient that you will do your best to find out the answers to their questions than to make something up on the spot which may turn out to be wrong. Nurses (and in particular specialist nurses) are a superb resource and oftentimes know far more about the condition than the junior members of the medical team, and may be able to spend more time with the patient than you can. Therefore, if possible try to have fellow healthcare professionals with you when breaking bad news.

Reference page

1.   Lalwani A. K. Current Diagnosis & Treatment, Otolaryngology Head and Neck Surgery, Second Edition, New York, McGraw-Hill, 2008

2.   Lee K. J. Essential Otolaryngology Head & Neck Surgery, Eighth Edition, New York, McGraw-Hill, 2003

3.   Cummings CW, Harker LA, Krause CJ, Richardson MA, Schuller DE, Krause CJ et al. Cummings Otolaryngology: Head and Neck Surgery Third Edition, St. Louis, Mosby, 1998

4.   Giles Warner, Andrea Burgess, Suresh Patel, Pablo Martinez-Devesa, Rogan Corbridge. Otolaryngology and Head and Neck Surgery, Oxford, Oxford University Press, 2009

CPSIA information can be obtained
at www.ICGtesting.com
Printed in the USA
LVHW05s1814030518
575858LV00014B/1565/P